When Demand exceeds Supply

When Demand exceeds Supply

The story of Caribbean Private Medical Education

Jorge C. Rios MD FACC, FACP

Library of Congress Control Number:		2016913267
ISBN:	Hardcover	978-1-5245-3363-2
	Softcover	978-1-5245-3362-5
	eBook	978-1-5245-3361-8

Print information available on the last page.

Rev. date: 08/18/2016

To order additional copies of this book, contact:
Xlibris
1-888-795-4274
www.Xlibris.com
Orders@Xlibris.com
745078

CONTENTS

ACKNOWLEDGMENTS

- To Barbara B. Rios, FACHE. Without her love and support, our Caribbean experience would not have happened, and without her editing of my writing, it would have read very differently
- To Shelly Winston, MHSA. Her ideas and editing helped make something better
- To Gregorio Koss, MD, FACC. He patiently read every word and made helpful notes

INTRODUCTION

THIS BOOK WILL discuss private medical education in the Caribbean. It will be presented from the perspective of a medical educator who developed experience at a well-known Caribbean medical school after having worked for three decades in allopathic medical schools in the United States.

I need to explain where I came from and what I did that gave me the experience to discuss the topic. This is not an autobiography, but a brief attempt to place Caribbean medical education in a proper perspective.

I graduated from the University of Buenos Aires Medical School in 1959. I experienced large class sizes, so what I saw in a Caribbean medical school did not come as a surprise. I had also observed large attrition. As it was said once in the *Chronicle of Higher Education*, Darwinian concepts apply to many Latin American universities, where attrition is the order of the day.

I completed my medical training in Washington, DC, and subsequently was on the faculty of Thomas Jefferson University and the George Washington University. In 1971 I returned to the George Washington University, where I progressed from assistant professor to the Eugene Meyer Professor of Medicine and Chair of the Department of Medicine (from 1976 to 1997), giving me experience with American medical education and the multiple issues of academic administration.

Upon my retirement in 2000 and after a brief period at the US Food and Drug Administration, I was offered to join Ross University School of Medicine, in the Commonwealth of Dominica, as executive dean. I have remained associated with Ross in several capacities until my recent and final retirement from teaching. During these many years, I taught thousands of medical students and personally advised and counseled hundreds of them. In the interim two Caribbean medical schools tried to recruit me. All of this gave me additional experience and information.

The work in both allopathic US schools and in Caribbean schools formed the background for my knowledge, experience, and opinions. I will like to share them without bias or prejudice. I hope that this book is of interest to faculty, department chairs, and deans of schools in the United States as well as to student applicants. They all may encounter facts about private medical schools in the Caribbean.

CHAPTER 1

Proprietary Medical Schools—an Overview

CARIBBEAN PROPRIETARY MEDICAL schools were established for one very good reason. Medical schools in the United States did not have an adequate capacity to meet the demands for physicians and were unable or unwilling to expand accordingly.

To understand why and how Caribbean schools started, it is important to review the factors that lead to their development and growth of these schools. The main factors include the following:

- Limited capacity of US medical schools and the insufficient number of graduates.
- Changing US population and increased demand for medical services by an older and wealthier society.
- The role of international medical graduates in compensating for the lack of US graduates. This allowed toincrease medical manpower without the cost of medical schools.

Once these issues are explained, it becomes clear why offshore proprietary medical education developed.

The looming physician shortage was simply a conflict between supply and demand.

For more than a quarter of a century, the number students graduating from US medical schools remained stagnant (table 1 and 2). This stagnation was accompanied by an explosion in the number of foreign medical graduates entering the United States, initially for residency training. This partially compensated for the manpower shortage, especially in hospitals.

Table 1-1. Number of Graduates, 1966–2008

1966	1981	1986	1992	1996	2000	2004	2008
7574	13634	16652	16427	15896	15716	15829	16268

Source: https://www.aamc.org/download/411782/data/2014_table1.pdf

Table 1-2. Number of Graduates from 1965 and 2015

Year	# Graduates	% Increase
1965	7574	
1975	13694	80%
1985	16117	17%
1995	15850	-1.60%
2005	15927	0.50%
2015	18075	11%

Source: https://www.aamc.org/download/411782/data/2014_table1.

It is quite apparent that from 1986 to 2008 the number of new graduates remained stable.

It is difficult to understand the rationale of policy makers who deprived qualified and motivated American citizens of obtaining a medical education while expanding the number of international graduates. They decided instead to bring many foreign graduates who had to return home after training due to visa requirements. This approach guaranteed a degree of medical services for the people while maintaining stable the number of new physicians.

The above facts appeared to have operated as a well-organized cartel. A *cartel* definition is "an agreement between competing firms to **reduce production using a variety of tactics**." This definition fits perfectly.

Organizations that controlled medical education managed, for whatever reason, to control production "using a variety of tactics"—in this case limiting access to medical school and limiting the number of physicians that graduated.

Medical education as it existed decades ago meets the definition of a cartel. Why a cartel? Having worked in US medical schools most of my adult life, I know that money, profit, and greed were not part of the academic medicine culture, and the reasons for such firm control on production quotas by US medical schools were not driven by greed or profits. So what other explanations can we rationalize?

- **Medical education is so demanding that schools needed to be very restrictive in admitting solely the highly academically qualified.** If that was the thought, it was obviously wrong. At the same time, thousands of foreign medical graduates were admitted whose academic credentials were not examined in great detail. Only a simple review of credentials and a standard examination by the Educational Council on Foreign Medical Graduates (ECFMG) and awarding a certificate were all that was needed for these graduates to start a residency in the United States. We can be sure that in many cases, their academic records were not comparable to some of the applicants not admitted to US medical schools.
- **Institutional inward thinking**. Individual institutions, mainly universities and medical schools, assessed their own internal needs (i.e., expansion of research, building new research facilities, clinical facilities, hospitals, etc.) without considering the perceived national issues that projected that a physician shortage was in the making.
- **Inaccurate projections of manpower needs.** Did the projections of a physician surplus (discussed later) derail any potential thoughts of medical school expansion?

- **The projection of physician needs may have been looked only at a regional or state level and not at the national level in aggregate.**
- **Universities may have feared expansion due to uncertain long term availability of federal and state funding.**
- **The frequent internal debates between the medical school and the university** that kept resources being directed to colleges at the expense of expanding the medical school, even if a physician shortage was looming at the distance.
- **The absence of federal government clear policies.** They had, during this period, serious concerns about physician manpower but did not impellent clear policies.

Some things did not make sense then or now! The United States limited the number of US citizens from attending and graduating from medical school while allowing an explosion of foreign physicians coming to the United States.

In a nutshell, the large difference between demand for physician services and the supply of new graduates is the main cause for growing shortage and the leading factor for the origin of Caribbean proprietary schools. As it happens in all areas of business, entrepreneurs recognized the needs of the market and developed a strategy to meet the needs.

The move to open medical schools in the Caribbean started in the 1970s and will be discussed in a different chapter. The creation of new schools has continued until today. The main problems with this growth were that it took place in foreign countries and there was minimal accreditation and regulation. It was a medical version of the gold rush!

One of my goals is to offer information and clarity regarding the quality of Caribbean education. There are excellent Caribbean schools as well as some very poor ones. Unfortunately, there have been major weaknesses in the accreditation system in the countries, and that has allowed some mediocre schools to exist.

The problem was simple. If you had the capital, all you had to do to start a new medical school was to reach a contractual agreement with a country, pass a local review by a locally appointed board, and go through a lax review by US authorities. Only in the last few years have accreditation systems—based on quality of education and outcomes, and utilizing practices common to United States and Europe—developed. Medical educational review and accreditation entities have been created but, so far, have accredited few schools. We hope that these accrediting bodies will elevate the quality of medical education similar to LCME in the United States.

To understand Caribbean medical schools and their role in American medicine, we need to start with a review of past and present issues regarding medical manpower.

Caribbean schools have been labeled "second-chance schools" since most of their students have applied one or several times to one or many US schools without success of admission. Several thousand students accepted the challenge to attend a Caribbean school and successfully graduated, completed a residency, and are now in practice. These schools not only gave them a second chance to become physicians but also demonstrated the imperfection of US schools admission exigencies. But before we proceed, we need to recognize the more than twenty thousand individuals who graduated from Caribbean schools and are now licensed physicians in the United States or Canada. They wanted to become physicians and were denied the opportunity by the limited capacity of US or Canadian schools. They had true grit to pursue their ambition, and they succeeded.

Caribbean medical schools have made a contribution to ease the physician shortage. They have especially impacted the shortage of primary care physicians. Despite their success, the leadership of academic medicine and some congressional leaders continue to oppose their existence and propose legislation to that effect. Pockets of resistance continue to exist both in academic medicine as well as political leaders. This attitude is often based on ignorance of facts or facts based on very old information when schools were just starting. They have failed to recognize the good schools from the bad ones and have grouped them together, often without even visiting them or auditing their educational quality.

Allow me to look at this issue as an educator whose responsibility was to help students to learn and succeed. Those who graduated and those who failed were given the same chances when they applied to a Caribbean school. Those who made it took advantage of the opportunity given and previously denied. Those who failed took a chance.

Those who failed are saddled with loans, and many try to find a reason and someone to blame. Unfortunately, they became victims of business operators who knew that many of these individuals had mediocre credentials and were very likely to fail and unlikely to graduate. They saw in each of them a way to increase their profit margin.

When schools report profits ranging from 20 to 50% of revenues, you fully understand that many student applicants were not looked as someone who deserves a second chance but as someone who will increase profit. They are the ones who provide the discussion grounds for those who believe that these schools are just profit-grabbing institutions, while those who graduate will argue vigorously that a Caribbean school "provided them the opportunity to fulfill their dream."

I will try to bring accurate information regarding Caribbean schools, identifying virtues and defects based on 2015 information and not on anecdotal, years-old data. We will try to discuss the issues in a fair and objective manner. I believe that my personal experience as an educator and academic administrator allowed me to develop a balanced view as well as an understanding of the issues of Caribbean or offshore medical schools.

CHAPTER 2

From Surplus to Shortage Do We Know How We Got Where We Are?

HOW DID WE get to where we are today? How did we get from reports suggesting that medical schools should decrease the number of students to the creation of several new schools all happening in thirty years?

In order to understand the reasons that have driven Caribbean Medical Education to the success it has enjoyed for four decades, we need to understand how the current physician shortage developed.

For many years, the shortage was developing, but it was concealed in part by the constant influx of foreign nationals graduated from foreign medical schools.

As years passed, physician manpower in the United States has undergone several periods, all of them gradually creating the physician shortage described today.

- The first period took place prior to World War II, when graduates from US medical schools constituted the very dominant group where the only practitioners. Physicians practiced mainly in their private office and some provided some pro bono work. There were no programs for the indigent or the poor, and city hospitals provided much-needed services for the elderly and the uninsured.

- The second phase occurred after World War II, which saw the arrival of a modest number of European physicians escaping the deprivation of the war.
- The third phase saw the arrival of foreign medical graduates, mainly from developing countries. This occurred because of the growing needs of physicians brought on by new hospitals and increased demand for services. The expansion of the J1 visa program allowed foreign physicians to enter the United States for residency training, and many of them stayed in the United States and obtained a license. This period is fascinating because it suggests that decisions were made, in good part, to protect the "exclusivity" of medical practice while ignoring needs of society.

  The number of US medical schools remained unchanged, and the enrollment capacity remained limited to the number previously established. No new medical schools opened for decades, and admission was restricted to a limited number of the best applicants in a very competitive process. The additional manpower needs were partially met through the admission of foreign national graduates from foreign schools who were allowed to train in the United States after passing and examination offered by the Educational Council for Foreign Medical Graduates (ECFMG). The examination, mandatory since 1960 in order to obtain a residence, provided a partial quality control since those who failed could not enter residency programs.
- The fourth phase was started when American citizens, unable to enter US medical schools, sought admission to foreign schools, mainly in Europe. This, again, is an incomprehensible event. The very limited capacity of medical schools left many qualified applicants without the chance of becoming a physician. At that time, a number of entrepreneurs recognized the difficulties many US citizens were experiencing entering a medical school and developed the idea to start schools in foreign countries, targeted mainly for US citizens. They started negotiating with Caribbean island governments with the goal of establishing

new medical schools dedicated mainly for those who had been denied admission to US schools.

- A sixth phase is happening now. Only recently, through the efforts of Jordan Cohen, MD, past president of the Association of American Medical Colleges (AAMC), efforts are underway to increase US medical school output and decrease dependency on international graduates. Recognition of the large physician shortage prompted the decision to expand class size in existing schools and also the creation of new medical schools. The goal was to increase the number of US graduates by 30% and therefore decrease opportunities of foreign graduates and US citizens studying medicine in the Caribbean.

The sequence of events described led to the serious shortage that should have been foreseen and acted upon earlier. In addition, the elitism of American academic medicine supported the belief that medical education had to be limited to few high academic achievers, thinking more on the individual merits instead of considering the population needs.

It appears that in each of these periods, there was a similar strategy. Limit the enrollment to US medical schools to the "best and the brightest" (experience showed that some were neither) and allow foreign physicians trained elsewhere to have access to the United States and correct the shortage.

All of the above gave the opportunity for these Caribbean schools to grow and expand and for investors to reap the financial benefit.

Estimating manpower needs is a complicated endeavor. It is a difficult and imprecise science. In theory, the number of medical school graduates should be in concordance with the number of physicians needed to provide comprehensive care to the population, continue active research, ensure a healthy and protected public and also to compensate for attrition caused by retirement and death of health-care providers. Unfortunately, multiple and ever-changing factors make projecting even more difficult. In addition, the education and training of a qualified physician requires approximately eight to twelve years and because of this long time frame, imprecise projections of US health manpower are made. The result is our current manpower predicament.

Other factors make forecasting very complicated. Who would have foreseen that forty years ago, changes such as physician productivity, the establishment of ancillary health-care staff, the prevalence of diseases (such as diabetes, obesity, HIV, etc.), and technological developments, as well as the complexity of methods used to treat and diagnose diseases.

Other important factors that influence the growing demand for services included the socioeconomic status of the population (better socioeconomic conditions is associated with higher expectations), or the creations of new federal and state programs. When Medicare and Medicaid were created, the demand for services increased. We are also seeing that the Affordable Care Act incorporates new subscribers and will again increase the demand for services. Factors that increase the demand for health services increase the need for more physicians.

As a the result of this complex problem, in the last thirty years we have seen manpower projections that evolved from a perceived critical surplus, as the Graduate Medical Education National Advisory Committee (GMENAC) and other reports indicated to the current belief of a dramatic shortage.

What were some of the conclusions predicting a physician surplus?

The GMENAC commission, created by the US government to evaluate issues with graduate medical education, indicated that by 1990 the number of physicians would reach 535,758, and they anticipated that the number of physician requirement was 374,800. GMENAC later recommended a physician supply of 466,000 (range 441,400–490,050). Revisiting the model in 1986, A. Tarlov, a highly respected academic internist and member of GMENAC, discussed in 1986, in an issue of *Health Affairs*, that the earlier forecasts underestimated what was likely to happen.

One of the major assumptions made by the GMENAC report was enrollment in new health maintenance organizations of an estimated 40% of the population. Major writers and researchers in the field supported these conclusions. The public however was reluctant to accept the HMO model and preferred the "open selection" option that existed.

As a result, enrollment did not meet materialize, as was anticipated and therefore, expectations of a surplus of physicians did not happen.

We have evolved from discussions of decreasing enrollment to the creation of new schools!

Now we are facing a physician shortage. Are the projections accurate? They are repeated with much conviction and quoted in newspapers throughout the United States and are now accepted as undisputable facts. This is guiding policy development.

At the request of the AAMC, in March 2015, a new study was released, "The Complexities of Physician Supply and Demand: Projections from 2013 to 2025." The study was performed for the AAMC by the company HIS, a large consulting firm. From that study, the AAMC indicated the following:

- Although physician supply is projected to increase modestly between 2013 and 2025, demand will grow more steeply.
- Total physician demand is projected to grow by up to 17 percent, with population aging and growth accounting for the majority.
- Full implementation of the Affordable Care Act accounts for about 2 percent of the projected growth in demand.
- By 2025, demand for physicians will exceed supply by a range of 46,000–90,000. The lower range of estimates would represent more aggressive changes secondary to the rapid growth in non-physician providers and widespread adoption of new payment and delivery models such as patient-centered medical homes (PCMHs) and accountable care organizations (ACOs).
- Total shortages in 2025 will vary by specialty grouping and include a shortfall of between
  - 12,500 and 31,100 primary care physicians; and
  - 28,200 and 63,700 non–primary care physicians, including
    - 5,100 to 12,300 medical specialists;
    - 23,100 to 31,600 surgical specialists; and
    - 2,400 to 20,200 other specialists.
- The physician shortage will persist under every likely scenario, including increased use of advanced practice nurses, greater

use of alternate settings such as retail clinics, delayed physician retirement, more physicians working part-time rapid changes in payment and delivery (e.g., ACOs, bundled payments), and other modeled scenarios.

Until now, the United States has dealt with physician manpower through a reliance on immigration policies, allowing a large number of foreign medical graduates to enter the United States. Recently however, some congressional leaders as well as representatives of organized medicine are attempting to cut the inflow of foreign medial graduates. The current approach has resulted in expanding of class sizes and the creation of several new medical schools in the United States as well as new osteopathic schools.

Let's hope these projections are accurate and that new discoveries, technological developments, or scientific breakthroughs previously unpredicted do not alter the needs and lead to a repeat of physician surplus or shortage.

CHAPTER 3

The US Population Growth and the Physician Shortage

THE GROWTH AND success of Caribbean medical schools is the result of the inadequacy of US medical schools to train the necessary number of physicians to meet the needs of the growing and aging US population. Graduates from Caribbean schools represent approximately 2% of practicing physicians (depending on geographic region) and have served to delay the crisis. Caribbean graduates as well as other foreign medical graduates are not enough.

Understanding trends in population growth and the causative factors of this growth will provide a better understanding on the current US needs for more physicians coming from US schools or recognized Caribbean schools. Graduates will be needed for many years even if sectors of US academia will continue to reject Caribbean graduates. It will be a long time before the AAMC recommendations on the number of physician graduates meet the needs of the US population and before the need for Caribbean graduates becomes unnecessary.

Reviewing some facts about the US population, the number of US physician numbers, their geographic distribution, age, and other factors that impact on adequate availability of physician services will lend support to the concepts expressed above.

Between 1980 and 2014, the number of physicians has grown by 23% while the US population has grown by 40%, and the ratio of physicians per thousand inhabitants has being dropping from 1.67 to 1.47, as shown in the table below. That data alone suggests that the physician shortage was in the making.

Table 3-1

Year	US Population	Population % Increase	Active MD	%MD Increase
1980	226,545,000		379,983	
		40%		**23%**
2014	318,816,000		468,942	

Source: https://www.census.gov/newsroom/cspan/1940census/

As a result of this population growth and the disproportionately slow expansion of the physician pool, the American Association of Medical Colleges has underscored the importance of the shortage of physicians. Their projection is that by 2025 the gap between supply and demand will be between 46,000 and 90,000 physicians. Similarly, a report by the Health Resources and Service Administration projects that the shortage would be about 55,100 by 2020.

Table 3-2

	2000	2005	2010	2015	2020
Supply	713800	764400	808100	842700	866400
Demand	713000	757000	805400	860600	921500
Difference	800	7400	2700	-17900	-55100

Source: http://bhpr.hrsa.gov/healthworkforce/supplydemand/medicine/physician 2020projections.

There are discrepancies in total number, but the fact remains that multiple organizations have anticipated this substantial shortages.

The number of physicians clearly has not kept pace with the growth of the US population, Can the population growth alone explain the current physician shortage? Unlikely. Other factors definitely impact the need for more physicians, including the following:

- Geographic distribution of physicians
- Aging of physicians

- Aging of the population
- Ethnic population changes
- Relationship between generalists and specialists
- The changes in medical practice and the use of technology
- The role of other allied health providers
- Society expectations of expanded medical treatment

We will review all them.

1. The geographic distribution of physicians enhances the issues created by physician shortage.

The ratio of physicians per 100,000 inhabitants vary among different areas of the country. Some large, underpopulated states with a low number of physicians are obviously magnifying and compounding the problems associated with the total shortage predicted.

The Health Resources and Services Administration has identified 6,100 areas with less than one primary care physician for every 3,500 people and estimate that the medical workforce would need over 8,000 additional physicians to address the shortage.

The number of physicians per 1,000,000 inhabitants is shown in this chart.

Fig. 3-1 Physicians per 100,000 (See table 1 for details.)

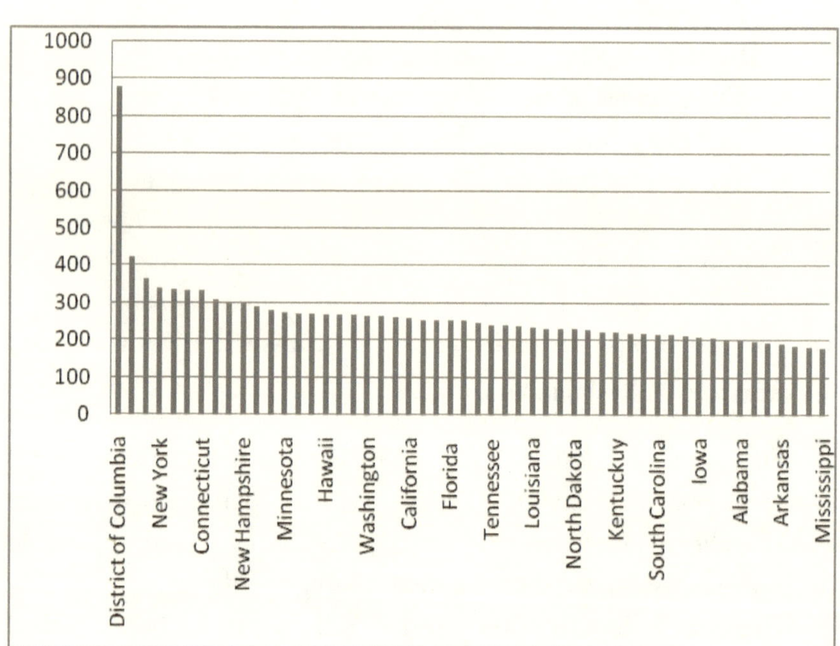

Source: American Medical Association Physician Masterfile

The above chart illustrates the uneven distribution of physicians in the United States. Some states have 40 percent less physicians than others, the largest numbers located in northeastern states (New York, Maryland, Connecticut) and the lowest numbers in southern and western states (Mississippi, Wyoming, Idaho). The District of Columbia appears to be out of proportion with the rest of the country, maybe as the result of the number of physicians working for the federal government in organizations such the military, the Department of Veterans Affairs, National Institutes of Health and other.

There are many reasons for the geographic maldistribution.

- Training programs are most often based in large urban centers, and 50 percent or more of the faculty practice in specialized fields. Trainees often follow the path of their trainers and mentors. This factor alone makes it less likely for physicians to settle in a rural area. As a consequence, the growth of specialization is a major contributor to the geographic maldistribution of physicians.

At the beginning of the twentieth century, physicians were nearly evenly distributed between rural and urban areas. In the intervening years, the specialization of medicine, the increasing social and professional isolation of rural areas, and growing economic disparity between urban and rural areas contributed to physician shortages in rural America.

- Life is different in urban and rural centers. Educational and entertainment availability in rural settings impacts quality of life as seen by many young physicians. Community factors such as inadequate schools for their children, fewer professional opportunities, and a paucity of cultural and other amenities for spouses and children play a large role in decisions not to locate or remain in rural areas. If high rates of poverty and extreme conditions are prevalent in the area, this can also make these areas unattractive to physicians.
- Another factor is the change in the number or women in medical school. Medical schools have now approximately a fifty-fifty female-male distribution. Physician gender is known to play a role in selection of practice location, particularly in nonmetropolitan HPSAs where female physicians are less likely to practice than male physicians. Traditionally, female physicians have been less willing than male physicians to practice in rural areas, although this trend appears be less sharp among recent graduates.
- **International medical graduates** somewhat alleviate the maldistribution. It has been shown that IMGs tend to practice in rural or underserved areas, in larger numbers than US graduates. IMGs disproportionately locate in high poverty areas of the largest US cities and also comprise a greater proportion of primary care physicians in designated rural shortage areas. Some waivers to the J-1 visas has helped place international medical graduates in underserved areas and have been found

to fill gaps in the physician workforce. Data in the practice preferences of Caribbean graduates is lacking, although we know that they enter primary care residencies in larger numbers than US graduates.

What could be done to decrease the problem of maldistribution, especially as it relates to graduates of Caribbean schools? The majority of medical students either in the United States or the Caribbean have to borrow money to pay for their education. A small percentage either have their own finances or relay on family help. The median debt level for a graduating medical student was $155,000 in 2008, with 25% of medical school students graduating with debt exceeding $200,000. Loan forgiveness plans as well as tax incentives are attractive alternatives for all students, regardless of where they graduate from, if they accept service in underserved areas.

2. Aging of Physicians

Another factor that will impact the physician shortage is the aging of physicians. The AMA Physician Masterfile of 2012, reports that 27.6% of 816,433 active physicians are 60 years of age or older. For the first time, the number of US physicians in their mid-50s (or older) has outpaced the number of physicians between the ages of 35 and 54. Retaining this physicians in some part time practice will be of help in handling the shortage. The data reflecting aging of physicians for the different states is shown in the next graph.

In a 2013 survey of over 20,000 physicians, the consulting company Deloitte noted that 62% indicate that "it is likely they will retire earlier than planned in the next one to three years. This perception is fairly uniform among all physicians, irrespective of age, gender, or medical specialty."

The Deloitte report also indicated that if physicians are not retiring outright, they will "scale back practice hours (55 percent) based on how the future of medicine is changing"

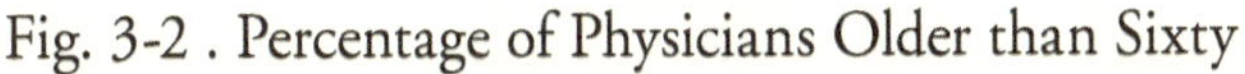

Fig. 3-2 . Percentage of Physicians Older than Sixty

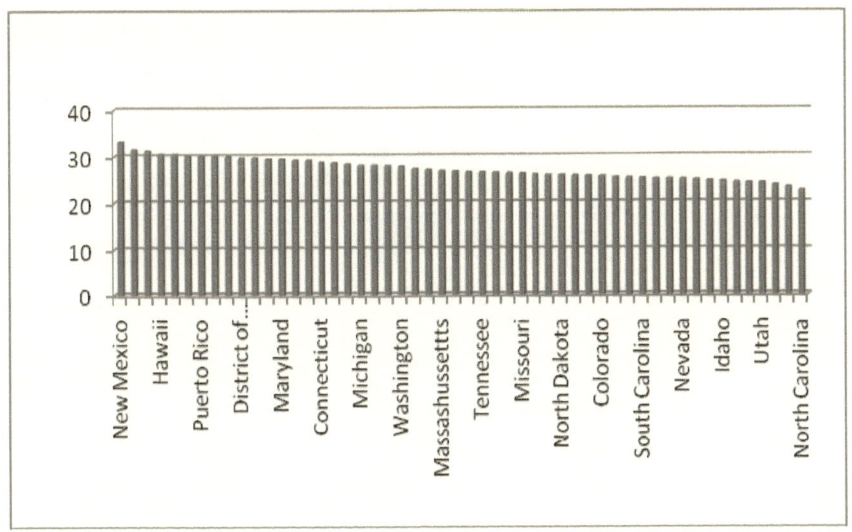

Assuming that physicians will retire between the ages of 65 and 70 one could conclude that just to maintain a balance in numbers, without correction of the existing shortages and population growth, more than 60,000 will have to enter the practice of medicine in the next few years. In 2014 AAMC reports that the class of 2014 had 18,057 graduating. This would suggest that with the current number of schools and its current of graduates per year, it may take years to correct the shortage caused by age alone. Graduates of offshore schools as well as IMGs remain essential to address the issue.

3. Aging of the Population

Aging of the population increases physician demand above the total population growth. What is the impact of population growth?

The growth of elderly population is shown in the enclosed graph.

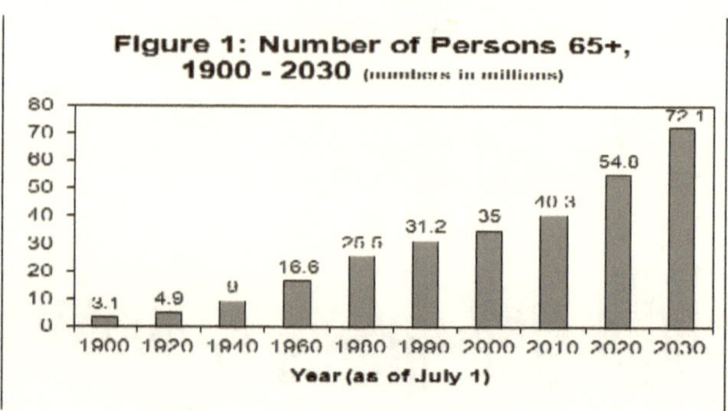

Source: www.ohsu.edu

The growth of the aging population, as shown above, will continue to result in a substantial increase in the demand for services. To demonstrate this point, we present the dramatic increase in the number of some procedures performed more often in older populations. Using data from the Agency for Healthcare Research and Quality, we show the increase over the recent years in some procedures, more commonly done in older populations. These examples demonstrate the increase in demand for services resulting from an aging population.

Table 3-3

	2000	2010	% Increase
Hip Replacements	165,000	302,839	82%
Knee Replacements	262,000	658,340	140%

4. Ethnic Changes in US Population

The choice of physician is influenced by the ethnic background of the patient. Studies in the United States has shown that both African Americans and Hispanics tend to seek physicians of the same cultural background. As shown in the following table, the populations in these two groups have grown much faster than the rest of the population. Physicians from these minority groups have increased only modestly. This gap exacerbates the perception of a major physician shortage.

Table 3-4

Race/Ethnic Group	1940	1960	2000	2010	1960 to 2010
Total Population	131,669,275	179,323,15	281,421,906	308,745,538	72%
White	118,214,870	158,831,732	211,460,626	223,553,265	41%
Black	12,865,518	18,871,831	34,658,190	38,929,319	108%
Hispanic (of any race)	2,021,820	5,814,784	35,305,810	50,477,594	768%
American Indian, Eskimo, and Aleut	333,969	551,669	2,475,956	2,932,248	778%
Asian and Pacific Islander	254,918	980,337	10,641,833	15,214,265	1460%
Some Other Race		87,606	15,359,073	19,107,368	
Two or More Races			6,826,228	9,009,073	

Source: http://www.infoplease.com/ipa/A0762156.html

Shortage of primary care physicians is common knowledge, and a shortage of specialists is also in the future. What the AAMC has shown is that primary care providers are not the only type of physicians that are going to be in shortage. The following are some of the published projections that I mentioned before but we consider important to cite again.

- Total physician demand is projected to grow by up to 17 percent.
- By 2025, demand for physicians will exceed supply by a range of 46,000 to 90,000.
- Total shortages in 2025 vary by specialty grouping and include A shortfall of between:
    - 12,500 and 31,100 primary care physicians; and
    - 28,200 and 63,700 non–primary care physicians, including

- 5,100 to 12,300 medical specialists;
- 23,100 to 31,600 surgical specialists; and
- 2,400 to 20,200 other specialties.

Caribbean graduates are providing relief. As will be shown in a subsequent section approximately 50% of graduates enter primary care residencies. We do not know, however, how many of them will pursue further fellowship training or, as indicated earlier, follow the trends of US graduates.

5. The Changes in Medical Practice and the Use of Technology

Medical practice has incorporated a number of technological procedures that necessitate specialized medical personnel and has, therefore, increased the need and demand for physicians and other health providers. The enclosed table shows the dramatic increase in modern technological procedures, all of which require specialized physician services.

Table 3- 5

	1995	2005	Increase
CT	24	85	254%
MRI	18	72	288%
PET	0	6	
All Types	42	163	288%

Some new technologies such as telemedicine allow expansion of service areas to larger parts of the country. The distance review by specialists of MRI, CT, and radiology are excellent examples of practices today that assist in the maldistribution of specialists. At the same time, new technologies demand physicians with new training while other services do not decrease.

6. The Role of Other Allied Health Providers

When the training of allied health-care providers became of age, hope was placed in that they would address the shortage of physicians by being extenders of primary care practices. This hope has only partially materialized since many physician assistants and nurse practitioners chose to leave primary care and work in different specialty areas. The chart below demonstrates that about 50% of both nurse practitioners as well as physician assistants are working in conjunction with specialists, and while it increases specialists' productivity, it fails to help the shortage of primary care providers.

Table 3- 6

Provider Type	Total	Percent Primary Care
Nurse Practitioners	106,073	52.0%
Physician Assistants	70,383	43.4%

Source: Agency for Health Care Research and Quality

7. Society Expectations of Medical Care

In January 2014, the Affordable Care Act extended access to health insurance coverage to an estimated 30 million previously uninsured people, resulting in an increased demand for physician services. For example, primary care providers will see, on average, 1.34 additional office visits per week, or a 3.8 percent increase of visits, nationally. The Ambulatory Care Act is expected to result in roughly 20.3 million additional primary care visits nationally and roughly 70 additional visits annually per primary care physician. These people will be newly insured through the marketplaces and account for more than a third of these visits. Emergency room visits by the newly insured are predicted to increase by 1.1 million, with those gaining Medicaid coverage accounting for more than two-thirds of these visits.

Most studies before passage of the Affordable Care Act projected shortages of at least 124,000 physicians by 2025, and there is general agreement that the additional 32 million covered lives that will result from the full implementation of the Affordable Care Act will require 31,000 new physicians.

In brief, the growth of the population, its increased ethnic diversity, the access to health care, and changing societal expectations are clear factors that explain and magnify the well-known physician shortage. In the absence of opportunities in US schools, those who feel the avocation to become physicians will continue to seek Caribbean schools to fulfill their goal.

CHAPTER 4

Foreign Medical Graduates and Physician Shortage

WHY ARE WE discussing foreign medical graduates? Foreign medical graduates were part of the historical development of medical manpower issues. They were the tool used to provide the essential manpower needs for hospitals and clinics while controlling and limiting the number of US graduates.

An AMA report defines *international medical graduate* in the United States as **"an individual who has graduated from a medical school outside of the United States or Canada."** As a consequence, US citizens graduated from Caribbean schools are included in these numbers a more meticulous and detailed analysis difficult.

The Educational Commission for Foreign Medical Graduates (ECFMG) is the entity charged to assesses the readiness of IMGs to enter accredited residency or fellowship programs in the United States regardless if they are US citizens or not.

In 2006, out of 902,053 physicians, 228,665 IMGs received medical degrees from 127 different countries, accounting for 25.3% of the total physician count. In a twenty-four-year period, non-IMG physicians grew by 91.4%, while IMGs increased by 170.2%.

In 2014 international medical graduates

- represent 22.7% of all physicians in the United States, 207,840 out of a total of 841,321 physicians with an active license;
- of these IMGs, 80% are involved in patient care and 16% are involved in academics; and

- they received medical degrees from 127 different countries, and the enclosed graph illustrates this point. In 2009, a total of 29,774 ECFMG certificates were issued for graduates from India, Dominica, Grenada, Pakistan, Netherlands Antilles, China, Philippines, Cayman Islands, Iran, and Israel. We need to note that graduates from Dominica and Grenada are graduates from Caribbean schools with an overwhelming number of US citizens. They are included in the total IMG pool, and in some topics, specific analysis become impossible.

Fig. 4-1. National Origin of IMGs.

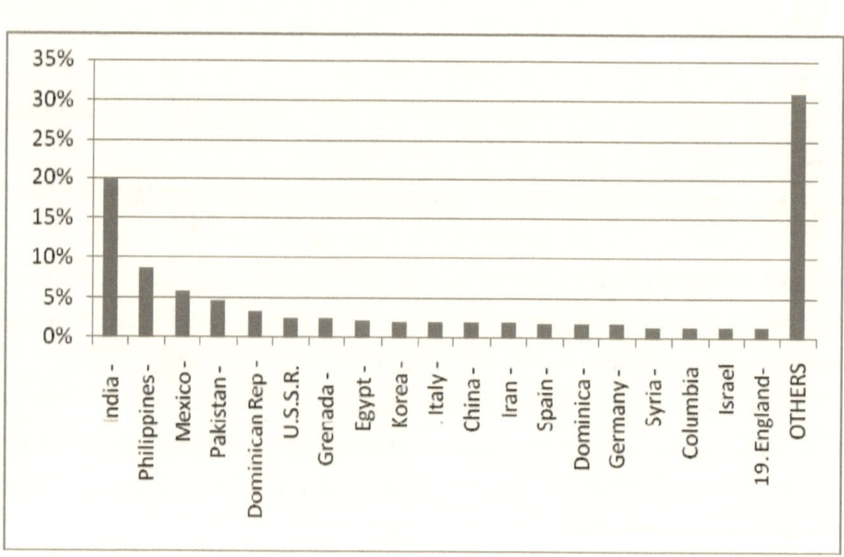

Source: http://www.ama-assn.org/ama/pub/about-ama/our-people/member-groups-sections/international-medical-graduates/imgs-in-united-state

Where are IMGs located?

The heaviest concentration of IMGs is in New Jersey (45% of physicians), New York (42%), Florida (37%), and Illinois (34%). The distribution in the United States is shown in the following graph.

Fig. 4-2

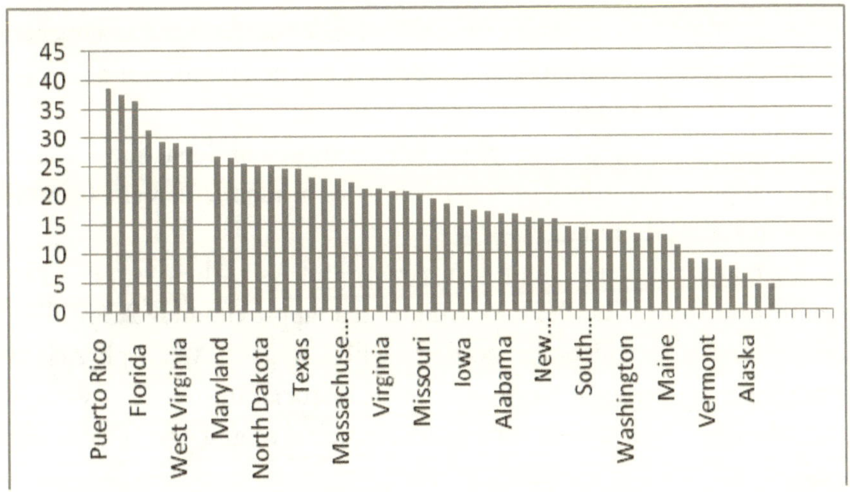

Source: http://www.ama-assn.org/ama/pub/about-ama/our-people/member-groups-sections/international-medical-graduates/imgs-in-united-state

The medical migration, caused by existing career opportunities in the United States and potential economic gains, resulted in a real brain drain to the countries involved.

Is this medical brain drain negative or positive? Is it appropriate for developed nations to guarantee their physician manpower by importing them from developing countries?

Western countries are doing the same with nurses, but the same is being done with other professions. This is a consequence of globalization of the economies. Should countries treat health professionals differently?

Medical education in many countries is heavily subsidized by the governments, and the United States is probably not spending enough government money in the training of more physicians. The poor developing countries lose their graduates without the return of service. Is that an ethical approach?

According to the World Health Organization (WHO), workers tend to go where the working conditions are best. While income is an important motivation, the sense of safety and job security the United States offers are important factors.

The United States is the land of opportunities. This is the most important factor for migration of physician, nurses, and all other professionals. Medical practice as well as academic medicine has opened its door to foreign graduates, and they have reached important positions in the academic ladder.

How many foreign-born physicians are deans or department chairs in developing countries? In most countries academic careers are well reserved for local graduates!

In many countries, mainly in Africa and Asia, there is a crisis in health workforce. The WHO estimates that approximately 2.3 million health service providers are needed to fill the gap. When physicians leave these countries, it has a significant financial impact. But what is the solution? Place a moratorium in physician migration? It does not make much sense or a realistic solution.

Remittance (the money that migrants earn working abroad and they send back to their home country) has been often mentioned as a gain to these countries. Unfortunately this will not solve the problem. It only obfuscates the issues. In many countries, remittance is a crucial source of foreign exchange. In 2004, global remittances to developing countries reached $160 billion, almost equal to foreign direct investments. A study focusing on physicians from the Philippines practicing overseas estimated that remittances were large enough to compensate for the economic losses associated with their emigration.

There is another issue not often discussed but equally realistic. Many developing countries, by subsidizing medical education have created an oversupply of physicians and other professionals. The graduate professional driving a taxi or having a severely underpaid job is a truth in many countries. Until the quality of life and job opportunities for professionals is improved in those countries, migration will continue. Don't blame the United States or other developed countries about physician migration when the problem is lack of opportunities for the local graduates. Look inside a developing country to determine what the problems are. Many countries have open access to medical school without considering manpower needs as a determining factor of class size. Some countries have created the migration issue by limiting opportunities to some of their most promising graduates.

Many experts believe that countries that recruit the most IMGs—the United States, Canada, United Kingdom, and Australia—have longstanding patterns of underinvestment in medical education and advocate for these countries to become more self-sufficient by adopting education policies with a goal of training a physician workforce close to the size of the demand for physicians in practice in their countries. The United States, through the AAMC and the LCME, have taken steps to increase the number of US medical graduates—in fact, with limited government intervention and limited federal funding.

In a global economy, there must be freedom of movement among workers, especially for highly trained professionals. Many countries—including Russia, India, and Philippines—have for-profit schools whose sole purpose is to train doctors for emigration around the world. These schools not only attract local students but a large number of international students. The rapid growth of medical schools in India, particularly private for-profit schools, is testament to the high interest in emigration.

Foreign citizens who are medical graduates enter the United States with different types of visas.

J-1 Exchange Visitor Program. The most common visa used to participate in US graduate medical education programs is sponsored by the Educational Commission on Foreign Medical Graduates. In order to obtain a J-1 visa an IMG must

- pass Step 1 and Step 2 of the United States Medical Licensing Examination (USMLE),
- obtaining a valid ECFMG certificate prior to the beginning of training (the Educational Council for Foreign Medical Graduates has to certify that the applicant has graduated from a recognized school and passed the licensing examinations), and
- hold a contract or an official letter of offer for a position in an accredited program of graduate medical education or training.

Upon completion of training, an IMG must either return to his or her home country for a period of two years before being eligible to return to the United States or obtain a waiver of this obligation. Under some circumstances, the two-year home residence requirement of the J-1 visa program can be waived. The individuals may find an interested governmental agency (IGA) to sponsor their waiver in exchange for agreeing to practice in an underserved area for at least three years. Waivers of J-1 visas can be obtained through the Conrad-30 Program, which allows sponsorship of up to thirty J-1 visa waivers per year.

Temporary Worker H-1B. The H-1B visa is for temporary workers in specialty occupations holding professional-level degrees, including graduates of foreign medical schools. The most common recipients of 1B visas are computer engineers and scientists. Unlike the J-1 visa, the H-1B visa does not have a two-year home residence requirement and allows a foreign national to remain in the United States for professional-level employment for up to six years. The current annual cap on the H-1B category is 65,000, with an additional 20,000 H-1B visas for foreign workers with a master's or higher-level degree from a US academic institution. Obtaining an H-1B visa has become increasingly difficult as the number of applicants in this category has increased considerably.

Immigrant Visas. IMGs may qualify for an immigrant visa (also known as a green card), which permits a foreign citizen to remain permanently in the United.

International medical graduates are a substantial component of the physician manpower in the United States. Without international medical graduates, the physician shortage would have become a critical issue several years ago. The following are some facts published in a very good monograph by the American College of Physicians that stated "contributions of International Medical Graduates IMGs are an important source of primary care physicians in rural and underserved areas." The following was abstracted from this monograph:

- About one quarter of community health centers rely on IMGs to fill physician vacancies.
- It has also been estimated that if all IMGs currently in primary care practice were removed, "one out of every five 'adequately served' nonmetropolitan counties would become underserved,

and the percentage of rural counties with physician shortages would rise to 44.4%."

- Critical access hospitals (CAH) in the United States rely heavily on IMGs, 60% of whom are internists.
- Over 50% of the nation's CAHs have or have had at least one IMG on the medical staff.
- IMGs make up more than half of the medical staff at 16% of CAHs.
- In addition, 62% of CAHs located in "persistent poverty" rural counties rely on one or more IMGs compared with 42% of rural counties that do not have a "persistent poverty" classification.
- A study in New York State revealed that the percentage of J-1 visa waiver IMGs planning to practice in shortage areas was triple that of US medical graduates.

At present, all international graduates (including graduates of Caribbean schools) must pass (Steps 1 and 2 of the USMLE). To the extent that this examination tests medical knowledge, they serve as quality equalizers, demonstrating the comparability between US graduates, Caribbean graduates, or those from other nationalities.

The following is data regarding passing rates for these two licensing examinations for foreign medical graduates.

Table 4-1

Step 1	% Passing
1st-Time Takers	77%
Repeaters	42%
Step 2- Clinical Knowledge	
1st-Time Takers	81%
Repeaters	45%
Step 2- Clinical Skills	
1st-Time Takers	73%
Repeaters	65%

Source: USMLE.org/performance data

Approximately, 95% of US schools' students pass these examinations, significantly higher than IMGs. Why such differences? It is easy to just say that itproves the educational differences. This is just a simplistic answer. When discussing IMGs, not Caribbean graduates, there are several possible explanations for these differences.

- First, cultural and language issues, the examination has a time limit, so it requires good English language skills to maintain a steady pace, otherwise the examination taker will not complete answering all questions.
- Second, inexperience with multiple-choice examinations. Many foreign schools conduct only oral examinations, and students have no practice with multiple choice questions, which require a certain strategy to complete on time.
- Third, takers of these examinations may have graduated several years before. US students take these licensing examinations while in medical school, while foreign graduates, on average, have been away from medical schools for three years.
- Fourth, the quality of medical education varies from country to country. Graduates from countries with a weak educational system are unlikely to pass the examination.

After graduation, and intended to train in the United States, foreign graduates enter the National Residency Matching Program (NRMP) in search of a residency. The number of FMGs entering the NRMP match has increased in the last few years, from 10,941 in 2010 to 12,467 2014, and they constitute 22% of the applicants registering for the NRMP match.

The success in securing a residency is low. The number matched is 49.8 as reported by the NRMP. For US citizens graduating from foreign schools, a comparable drop has been noted, from 53% in 2010 to 47.3% in 2014. This will be discussed in greater details in a different chapter.

After completing residency, IMGs will locate anywhere for practice. The geographic distribution of foreign medical graduates and where they enter practice is shown in the enclosed chart. There is evidence that IMGs will tend toward practicing in rural and underserved areas, definitely higher than US graduates. The trend is not sufficient to correct the problem affecting rural medicine. The reasons for the trend of IMGs to practice in underserved areas is not known but probably related to lower number of practitioners and better practice opportunities.

Fig. 4-3. Geographic Distribution of IMGs 2012

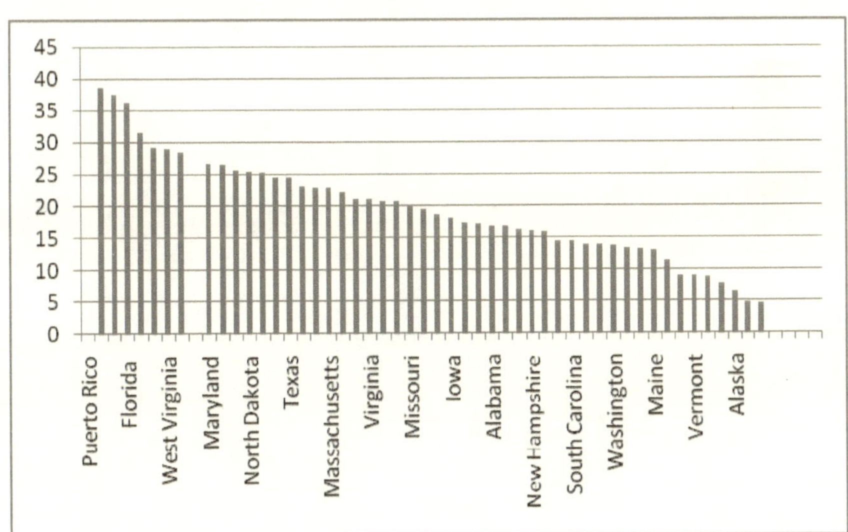

Source: http://www.ama-assn.org/ama/pub/about-ama/our-people/member-groups-sections/international-medical-graduates/imgs-in-united-state

It is should be clear that the shortage of physicians in the United States would be of catastrophic proportions without IMGs. The shortage is alleviated only by the number of IMGs who continue to enter the system. Another example of the importance of IMGs to physician manpower is that approximately 7,000 of the 25,000 residents who complete a US residency are foreign medical graduates. The system was designed with heavy reliance on IMGs. That was and is the way, and now they realize that it has to change.

All the information presented above explains and highlights the magnitude of the issues and its causes. All IMGs as well as Caribbean school graduates (considered as IMGs) are a response to a flawed system created and implemented decades ago.

Now is time to talk about Caribbean proprietary schools.

CHAPTER 5

Caribbean Schools

CARIBBEAN COUNTRIES HAVE a long history in medical education that started in the sixteenth century with the Universidad Autónoma de Santo Domingo. This is an impressive history, especially since many of the schools in Europe only started in the fifteenth century and the oldest, the University of Bologna, started in the eleventh century. The first medical school in the United States, the University of Pennsylvania, was founded in 1765.

Until 1978, existing schools were regional schools, devoted mainly to students from the Caribbean community. The concept of offshore schools, almost exclusively dedicated to US and Canadian students, had not fully developed yet. A small number of US students entered these Caribbean regional schools, but those who decided to go to medical school abroad did it mainly in Europe.

Caribbean schools and universities could be divided in two groups, regional and offshore.

Regional Universities

Until the advent of proprietary education, all Caribbean schools mainly served citizens of Caribbean countries although they sometime accepted few US citizens. Some of these universities have long histories and deserve mention.

- The **Universidad Autónoma de Santo Domingo** has been in existence since 1538. It started as the University of Santo Tomás de Aquino and was created on October 28, 1538, by means of the papal bull *In apostolatus culmine.* The new university was organized in four schools: medicine, law, theology, and arts.

In the year 1801, as a consequence of the Haitian occupation of the country, the university ceased operating. It was not reopened until 1815, when Spain resumed control of the island.

- The **Universidad de La Habana** is the oldest university in Cuba, established in 1728, originally as a religious institution offering programs in fields of natural sciences, social sciences, and humanities. It was first called **Real y Pontificia Universidad de San Gerónimo de La Habana**, and it was authorized by King Philip V of Spain. In 1952, when Fulgencio Batista took power, the university became a center of antigovernment protests, and the dictator closed the university in 1956. After Fidel Castro took power, they attempted to eliminate antirevolutionary ideas.
- The **Faculty of Medicine of the State University of Haiti** has functioned since 1867 and is located in Port-au-Prince. Its origins date to the 1820s, when colleges of medicine and law were established. In 1942 the various faculties merged into the University of Haiti. In 1960, Duvalier's government controlled the university and renamed it the State University of Haiti. The university's independent status was confirmed in the Haitian constitution of 1987.
- **The University of the West Indies** operated its school of medicine since 1948 and is, at present, the premier regional university for Caribbean countries. The university was founded in 1948, on the recommendation of the Asquith Commission, established in 1943 to review higher education in the British colonies. Initially it had a special relationship with the University of London as the University College of the West Indies (UCWI). The university college achieved independent university status in 1962. The Saint Augustine Campus in Trinidad, formerly the Imperial College of Tropical Agriculture (ICTA), was established in 1960, followed by the Cave Hill Campus in Barbados in 1963.

- Cuba, since the revolution that brought Castro to power, has made health care an important element of its foreign policy. Either Cuban physicians traveled to foreign countries on missions or students from developing countries were given scholarships to study medicine in Cuba. One excellent example is the formerly called **Escuela Latinoamericana de Ciencias Médicas**, established in 1999 and operated by the Cuban government. ELAM has been described as possibly being the largest medical school in the world, with an enrollment with approximately 19,550 students from 110 countries as reported in 2013. All those enrolled are from outside Cuba and mainly come from Latin America, Africa, Asia, and the Caribbean. The school accepts students from the United States.

  The school of medicine is officially recognized by the Educational Commission for Foreign Medical Graduates (ECFMG) and the World Health Organization and is fully accredited by the Medical Board of California. ELAM was an idea by Fidel Castro, as part of efforts to transport influence and political principles to other regions. This policy was known as the Integral Health Plan for Central America and the Caribbean.

  ELAM accepted ten US students in 2001 and was classified by the US government as a cultural exchange to avoid the restrictions of the US embargo.

Off-Shore Proprietary Schools

These schools, all of them for profit, were created to attract US and Canadian students who could not obtain admissions to US or Canadian medical schools.

As indicated earlier, the reasons for starting these schools was a response to very obvious market needs. Thousands of American students who wanted to attend US schools could not be admitted because the capacity was limited and the demand much greater than the supply. The early trend was for students to go to European schools. Distance, language, and duration of education made this option less attractive.

These circumstances provided an opportunity for creative entrepreneurs to negotiate with different island governments to open new medical schools. Proprietary schools locating themselves in a Caribbean island were close to the mainland, the local language was English, and the operating costs were lower than in the United States or Europe. Above all, they correctly perceived that there was a great demand for medical education. These schools had and continue to have only one mission: to teach students to pass US licensing examinations and graduate. They have no research ,conduct no laboratory resesearch and they are not active on clinical research. They do not operate their own residency programs or hospitals and admit students more than one class a year, commonly three. These features minimize cost and enhance potential profit. It represented a bonanza for investors.

The starting of the schools was adventurous, especially for the students. All schools had common features.

- They recruited US students wcould not gain acceptance in US schools. The initial group of students saw these schools as their last opportunity, and they were willing to take a risk with a school of unknown quality. They were dedicated and ambitious. Hearing some of their stories, you have no choice but to admire their resiliency. The school was unknown, the facilities primitive. It is reported that one school started with one cadaver in a bathtub and classes were conducted in a hotel. Students had to quickly adapt to a new culture, food was local, and none of the American niceties were available. The weather could be horrendous during the rainy season, and if a hurricane hit (as it did), destruction was such that they could not find places to stay. Despite all of these mishaps, the tellers of the stories endured all the discomfort, and with true, pure grit, they proceeded. Some of these individuals are today successful practitioners.
- The entrepreneurs that planned these schools, searched until they found a Caribbean island government receptive to the idea and would give them a home. The islands were perfect

sites for their plan. All these islands are in relative proximity to the mainland United States and had airline connections to several large cities, directly or through San Juan, PR. Since most schools created no housing for students, they had to rent from locals as well as buy necessities from locals. That created new construction opportunities for apartments and would give the population sources of income and work. The government would collect much needed tax revenues. For local governments it represented a new source of foreign investment and new source of employment for its citizens.

- The school owners would incorporate overseas and avoid paying US taxes. Everyone gained.
- They all started in a small way. Starting a medical school in a temporary building was no surprise. Gradually they expanded, and some offer today large and complex medical school campuses with up-to-date technology.
- At the beginning, classrooms were small, mainly a room with tables, chairs, a projector, and a projecting screen. Anatomy laboratories were primitive and the library modest. Since then, schools built comfortable auditoriums and classrooms. In some, outstanding audiovisual and information technology has been installed.
- The dominant method of education at the time was classroom lectures. One professor could teach a class of fifty or a class of three hundred and repeat the topic three times a year to new classes. At the beginning, some academic departments had a faculty of one or two!
- Bringing three classes a year maximized the work output of the faculty, creating a high ratio of revenues over expenses. This model continues today and explains the financial success of the schools.
- As discussed elsewhere, large number of the faculty members came from different countries, that included few retired Americans or Canadians and others from all over the world. This kept salaries at minimum and affordable.

- The facilities, office, and library were often in temporary buildings that were later replaced by modern facilities with comfort and elegance.
- The administrative staff was recruited among locals, with substantial savings in salaries since they were paid in local currency.

A consulting study done for the World Bank, to be discussed later, reviewed these plans and concluded that private medical education was indeed a very profitable business.

These initial steps in the late 1970s saw the starting of three schools, and they represented the beginning of offshore medical education.

The initial results were less than outstanding and created, in the minds of American medical educators, the impression of low-quality education offered by greedy investors. As years passed, several schools improved quality, staffing, and facilities, and added modern and excellent technology. Today some offer educational outcomes comparable to some US medical schools.

Almost forty years have passed since the first schools started. Since then more than twenty schools have opened, some as recent as 2007. For many years the medical establishment, especially academic medicine, looked at the graduates with disdain, and some still refuse to consider any of them for residency positions regardless of what Caribbean school they graduated from.

The incongruency of such a position is difficult to comprehend today. I will be the first to recognize that while there are some very good Caribbean schools, there are several at the other end of the spectrum, and if the accreditation process was rigorous and centralized, some would not be accredited.

Several questions could be asked.

How and who can we make that determination of which school should be allowed to operate and which should not?

Does that judgment apply to all its graduates? For example, should a student who scores 300 on Step 1 be discriminated against because of having attended a school that people think is bad, or should he be judged on his merits?

Can we also say that a graduate of one of the Caribbean schools is always worse than a graduate of any US medical schools?

What parameters do we use to make such a potentially discriminatory judgment? Do we judge the individual or the school?

What parameters could we use to evaluate a Caribbean school and also compare them to the performance of some US school? The ones listed below could be a good start.

- ➢ Mean Step 1 scores for one year
- ➢ Mean Step 2 scores for one year
- ➢ Graduation rate—ECFMG certificates obtained in one year NRMP match outcome—percentage of graduates who obtain a residency through the match or outside the match
- ➢ Faculty student ratio in basic sciences
- ➢ Faculty student ratio in clinical sciences
- ➢ Facilities and technology
- ➢ Student support services
- ➢ School educational technology

The constant issue is how to formulate an opinion regarding a school when there is no source of centralized and verified data and information. Is the source of the data credible and can that data be confirmed and validated?

For example, some schools will inform that 90% of students passed Step 1 on the first trial. What is the denominator? How is the percentage calculated? Is it 90% of one group of students in one academic year? Is it 90% of all students taking the examination during one, two, or three years, and not just a selected data point?

One of the important issues with Caribbean schools is the inability to validate data. As opposed to US schools where the AAMC is the repository of data and, when published, it represents data for all schools reporting, there is no such data repository for Caribbean schools, and the presentation of data is left to individual schools and often incorporated into websites or marketing material.

The most critical statistic is the number of graduates per year. That is available from the ECFMG. A ratio of graduating students over the number of students that registered at the school would give everyone statistics regarding graduation rate and, correspondingly, attrition. That is critical information.

In 2014, doctors Lynn Eckert, MD, and M. van Zanten, PhD, from the Foundation for Advancement of International Medical Education and Research published a report that discusses Caribbean proprietary education and includes the number of certificates issued by the ECFMG, an indicator of how many students are graduating in one year.

In 2013, ECFMG issued 3,240 certificates. As shown in the enclosed table, 2,490 (or 74%) came from the five schools listed below.

Table 5-1

American University of Antigua	347
American University of the Caribbean	281
Ross University	815
St George's University	891
Saba University School of Medicine	156

The remaining 750 ECFMG certificates were given by the all the remaining schools.

It should be noted that in 2013 DeVry (who owns booth Ross University and the American University of the Caribbean) graduated 1,096 students, or 34%. One of every three of all graduates of Caribbean schools who received an ECFMG certificate graduated from a school owned by DeVry, who has become the major force in Caribbean medical education.

Many Caribbean school have facilities and technology that are quite comparable and sometimes superior to US schools. This has evolved over time. Some examples of techology available on some of the campuses includes video conferencing, wireless availability throughout the campus, electronic libraries with all needed texts, computerized examination centers, multiple TV monitors in each classroom, and many others.

Some brief information regarding the different schools is found in appendix 4.

In the following chapters, we will address different topics regarding education in Caribbean medical schools.

CHAPTER 6

Cost of Education

THE COST OF medical education remains a major concern to students and families. People constantly ask why is that college or professional schools tuition has continued to go up every year. The issues are many, and as I was told many years ago by a patient, a former secretary of the treasury, "Education is like health care, the consumer receives no information to explain the reasons for either the cost or the increases in tuition, but since the money is borrowed long-term, it has no immediate effect on the individual."

According to data provided by the Labor Department, the cost of education has increased by 200% from 1985 and 2005, The most dramatic increase however, occurred between 2005 and 2015, when it went up another 35% percent with a total increase from 1985 until 2015 of 550%. As a point of comparison, the cost of medical care has gone up 300% and the consumer price index increased by 100%.

Table 6-1

% Increase from 1985	
Education	550%
Medical Care	300%
Gasoline	200%
Shelter	120%
Consume Price Index	110%

This issue has finally risen to the front of public discussions during the 2016 presidential campaign. Unfortunately, politicians are more interested in finding ways to increase financial support and spend more money than to look at the reasons why costs are out of control and try to propose and create suggestions and alternatives.

As an example, for academic years 2015–2016, the tuition in a US private school ranges from 47,160 to 57,136 dollars. As a result, borrowing to finance education continues to go up, much higher than the increase cost on health care, and many students find education unaffordable. There has to be reasons as to why neither hospital nor schools can ever explain or show you where the costs are coming from in a detailed billing statement.

Efforts are being made, with a modicum of success, to control the increasing cost of health care with programs such as managed care and similar variants. Similar efforts are needed in education, first, to understand the continuous incremental cost of education and, second, to bring the cost of education under control. Unfortunately the laws of the market do not operate freely neither in education nor in health care. Competition will come sooner or later and start bringing reality into the issue. Caribbean medical education that is nothing more than an extension of American education funded in part by the US government through student financial aid is very similar.

What Are the Prices of Medical Education in the Caribbean?

The following table lists tuition prices (2015) in asscending order for some of the well knownCaribbean schools.

SABA UNIVERSITY..$119,825

AMERICAN UNIVERSSITY OF THE CARIBBEAN..... $179,850

ROSS UNIVERSITY... $187,900

ST GEORGES UNIVERSITY.. $233,733

Some schools are reported to have much lower tuitions, as low as approximately 10,000 dollars a year.

Are all these schools omparable? We will report on how to evaluate but essentially, it has to be on outcomes of education although the quality of the facilities and the student support needs to be taken into consideration.

Looking at the reported tuition for Caribbean medical schools, we can see great differences. It is curious that the schools whose students are eligible for US financial aid are among the most expensive. We are not questioning that they are perceived as the best schools. Have they demonstrated the reasons why their tuition is what it is, or is just coincidence.

Since, as opposed to US schools, Caribbean schools have only one source of funding—student tuition—they could be able to provide a clear explanation of cost. The Department of Education would appreciate that information!

Tuitions ranging between for those extremes forces us to ask some questions.

- Is the education comparable?
- Are the facilities comparable?
- Are the outcomes (Step 1, Step 2, graduation, residency match) comparable?
- Are there some licensing issues? How many states will grant the graduate a license to practice medicine in all 50states. There some states that do not recognize the degree given by some schools.
- What percentage of tuition is spent on marketing and recruitment? What is the ratio between instruction cost and marketing cost?
- What is the profit margin for all these schools?

US schools have multiple sources of income such as research overhead, clinical practice income, endowments, and donations and, therefore, are in a position to create multiple internal subsidies. This can lead to some internal conflicts.

Caribbean schools are almost exclusively supported by tuition, so a clear explanation of cost could be done. In some cases, revenues form medical school tuition subsidize the operational cost of less profitable ventures or colleges.

Opening a medical school in the Caribbean has had distinct advantages from a business perspective, and it is a very profitable venture. In 2004 a report was submitted to the World Bank by the group Swedish Development Advisers that analyzed Caribbean education.

They stated

> It is significantly less expensive and easier to establish an offshore medical school in the Caribbean. The low threshold for founding offshore schools is both positive and negative as the initial cost is low, but that competition is high as more and more offshore schools open. The low threshold is mainly due to the following:
>
> x Lower standards for accreditation enforced by local accreditation agencies,
>
> x Medical or basic research is not required for accreditation nor carried out voluntarily by the offshore schools, and
>
> x Salaries are usually lower than US schools
>
> The schools in the Caribbean are founded by physicians and entrepreneurs with the motive to eventually reap a profit from the schools. Although none of the offshore medical schools were willing to provide financial statements, it is likely that basic teaching is highly profitable and was estimated at 29%.

This report highlighted how things were in 2004. What has change since then to 2015?

The accreditation process has improved dramatically, and the good schools offer levels of education and facilities comparable or similar to many US schools. On the other hand, the opportunity persists for entrepreneurs to find a place in the Caribbean to open a medical school and start marketing offering lower tuition. Consumers must be aware!

As indicated in the report to the World Bank mentioned above, **medical education in the Caribbean is a highly profitable business**. There are several clear reasons why.

- US **taxes.** Many schools are incorporated overseas, so they avoid paying US corporate taxes. **Local taxes and custom taxes** are often waived or agreed at a preferential rate. These beneficial tax agreements are made to entice the investors to open the school in that country. From the country perspective, this is a reasonable view. Small Caribbean countries have limited economies and have depended on agriculture and tourism as the economic pillars. A medical school brings employment and consumption and becomes critical to the gross domestic product of the country. Many of these countries were in economic difficulties, and they were helped by the increased consumption brought by faculty and students. Many have implemented a value added tax on most purchases applicable to everyone in the country. This has helped to generate additional local tax revenue.
- **Staff salaries** for local employees are paid in local currency and are significantly lower than US wages. For example, the minimum wage in some countries that house medical schools is the equivalent to 1.5 US per hour compared to $7.25 per hour in the United States.
- **Faculty salaries.** The best Caribbean schools are starting to pay competitive salaries when compared with US schools and can hire US or Canadian faculty, many of them retired, from very reputable schools or can hire young PhDs having just completed their postdoctoral period.

  One of the factors why working abroad is advantageous to both the school and the US faculty are the tax advantages. As it will be discussed in a separate chapter, US expatriates do not pay income taxes in the United States on the first 100,800 dollars (for 2015) and adjusted annualy for inflation and pay no local income tax.

Many of the schools have even cheaper ways to operate. They mainly recruit faculty from developing countries at much lower salaries, sometimes as low as $50,000. We are not disputing faculty competence but simply indicating that they have lower salary expectations than US or Canadian faculty.

- Another issue associated with cost is the student-to-faculty ratio. As indicated in the report to the World Bank mentioned above, US schools have a student-to-faculty ratio averaging close to 4:1. Caribbean schools' faculty-student ratio ranges between 9:1 to 13:1. The combination of lower faculty salaries, faculty teaching the same classes three times a year, and a lower number of faculty are substantial contributors to the high profit margin.
- Other advantage are the much lower legal costs as well as the cost of staff fringe benefits.

All of these advantages make the cost per medical student substantially lower than in US schools.

There are areas were Caribbean schools have expenses not commonly incurred by US schools, and one of this is clinical education. US schools have not paid for their students to train in US hospitals. In most cases, Caribbean schools have to pay for clinical education. Schools sign contracts with hospitals, as will be discussed later, and pay a certain amount per student per week. The increased competition to obtain sites to train their medical students has resulted in an increase in the amount per student that hospitals or clinics receive. The reported figure reaches $500 per student. Examples: as media reports indicate, St. Georges signed an agreement with New York hospitals for $100 million to train medical students, and Ross has signed a $25 million ten-year contract with Kern Medical in California for the same purpose.

By far, a major difference with US schools is the cost of marketing. US schools do not have that expense (they may have it for the hospital and clinic) but not for student recruitment. Offshore schools spend a lot of money in advertising, marketing, and recruitment. The competition is fierce and every marketing technique is used. It is impossible to establish what percentage of student tuition is spent on marketing and recruiting of new students.

Corporate profits are a percentage of tuition and is maintained a secret. Since most schools are privately owned and often operate as a foreign corporation, they do not have to report profits. Anecdotal information says that it can be as high as 50%.

It is clear, however, that the advantages must overpower the disadvantages and the profit margin must be high, as highlighted in the 2004 report to the World Bank mentioned earlier.

If one wants to do a comparison of tuition of Caribbean schools, it must be done strictly with private US schools that do not receive state funding.

An equally difficult analysis to perform is cost (tuition) versus outcomes. These differences may not be significant when comparing to US schools since they all are accredited by the same body. Differences among US schools are more based on research funding or the very soft criteria of school reputation.

What about Caribbean schools? How does one evaluate the benefits of a Caribbean education comparing different schools?

Tangible benefits in quality of education need to be correlated against tuition. Some basic parameters that will give information regarding the quality of education and the future chances of success after graduation include the following:

- USMLE Step 1 and Step 2 scores. This should include not only the percentage of students passing the examinations but the mean passing score for a given class in a given school. This is an important parameter because score are linked to the probability of obtaining a residency position.
- The percentage of students who get a residency through the National Residency Matching Program.
- Reputation. A very difficult concept to define. From all available reports, St. Georges in Granada and Ross in Dominica appear with the longest history and reports of the highest reputation.

The problem with Caribbean schools' information is that they are not reported by any independent organization. The information should be made readily available, and it should be the responsibility of an organization that accredits schools to do so.

At the moment the only information available come from the schools themselves, usually incorporated in their marketing material. It would be important to have more credible centralized information, especially if we look at the debts that students will incur.

As we will discuss later, the US government should take an active role in addressing the issue of cost and quality of education, especially for schools eligible for US financial aid. They should monitor Step 1 scores, timely completion, and graduation rates, and link it to loans and loan amounts. It is clear that tax dollars are a substantial role of the income of private medical schools and the Department of Education should be very proactive in this area. For those foreign schools not receiving US financial aid, the accrediting bodies should expand their role.

CHAPTER 7

Class Size, Graduation, and Attrition

CLASS SIZE, GRADUATION rates, and attrition are perhaps the most commonly asked questions in any conversation about Caribbean medical education. In this chapter we will discuss these topics using available data regarding the group of proprietary Caribbean medical schools and not using any data from a specific school. We will do that because, as mentioned before, there is no single source to verify specific data, and data is presented by the schools from a marketing perspective with recruitment intent.

Class Size

The reputation is there. Any search conducted will tell you about the large class size of Caribbean schools. The days of schools starting with eight to ten students are over. Schools reporting very small classes are usually new, starting schools.

Class sizes vary from school to school, and it is very difficult to get an official number. The data comes mainly from student sites. However, I know of 500 or more students in a couple of schools and also of small classes of 50 or less students in the smaller, less well-known schools. If teaching uses classroom lectures as the prevalent didactic method, class size is less important. I have seen, in a US school, a classroom with 200 students, when medical students and physician assistant students attend a combined course. At present, US schools have expanded class size, and an entering class of 190 students is not uncommon.

As discussed in a different chapter, class size is likely to vary from semester to semester as a result of marketing and recruiting efforts.

Information on class size is sometimes obtainable from student blogs. One of them (*Medical School Success*) indicated the following:

> The class sizes per trimester for the top Caribbean medical schools are listed below:
>
> - St. George Medical School: 400
> - AUC Medical School: 100–200
> - Saba Medical School: 80–100
> - Ross Medical School: 400–600

Based on personal observations, these numbers appear accurate. In schools with three semesters, the September class will be the largest because it captures students who graduated from college in May, so the school will have a larger applicant pool. Among faculty members it is common knowledge that the incoming May class can be the weakest, and therefore, admission criteria will be as low as you can accept. There is no consistency in admission criteria from semester to semester, just get enough students in to meet budget.

The problems with class size do not come in the first semester. It comes later, when lecture is no longer the principal method of teaching and the move to clinical teaching or a hospital clinical settings, where groups of eight to ten is the maximum you should have for a meaningful education. Any more makes the clinical teaching difficult, and rooms could be overcrowded. That transition is complicated because it necessitates a large enough faculty with clinical skills to absorb the large number of groups that need to be created. That is one of the main difficulties. At Caribbean schools, to teach any clinical medicine, you either have clinical faculty members teaching many large groups or large overcrowded groups, and neither one is good. So the real issue is not how many students you have in a classroom at the beginning of medical school, but do you have the resources you need to create quality clinical teaching? If we pursue this further, accrediting bodies should determine that incoming new classes should be no more than the average number of clinical students plus the calculated attrition. No doubt, this will have an impact on finances, but it will go a long way toward consistency in educational quality.

Many schools are decreasing the number of classroom teaching hours evolving to a system approach incorporating small group teaching starting from the first year of school. Adequate number of faculty must be available from the very start of school. And that has an impact on total faculty size.

Attrition

A definition of attrition is necessary so we can compare outcomes in different educational institutions. For example:

- What percentage of students, enrolling at a specific date graduate at the end of four years?
- What percentage of students graduate in 5 or 6 years?
- What is the number of students failing school for academic reasons?
- How many leave for nonacademic reasons?

  Detractors of Caribbean education are prompt to indicate that the high attrition is clear evidence of greed and the desire of high profits. This view has a good foundation. It is difficult to think other reasons to explain entering classes of 500 students that graduate 300! Either student selection and admission criteria are weak or that high attrition will leave many with loans to repay.

There are many factors that lead to attrition:

- Realization that the student made a wrong career choice or the wrong school choice
- Academic failures and realization that they could not cope with the material
- Personal, behavioral, and psychological issues
- Health

- Transfer to another school (often to a less rigorous Caribbean school, rarely to a US school)

The common point of comparison for everyone is the attrition rate in US medical schools, where it is commonl to be 3%. These numbers have changed.

The AAMC reported in 2014 that for the period 2009–2010 that

- eighty one percent (81%) of medical students, not concurrently working on another degree, completed their medical education in four years;
- in the same period, 94.1% graduate in five years; and
- reasons for this are not clear but often related to desires of having a "good quality of life period" in the middle of medical school.

What is the Caribbean data?

Whatever little information is obtained has to be drawn from informal sources and not from the schools. After reading many blogs written by students, the best we can surmise is that

- attrition ranges from 10% to about 30%, and
- graduation is not higher than 60% to 70% in up to six years.

As mentioned above, the factors that influence attrition are multiple, but the most frequent one is academic failing, followed by personal issues and financial problems, debt, loans, and othersetc. Transfer—most commonly to another, usually easier—school (by weak or failing students) and rarely to a US school.

That is why a serious discussion about attrition is necessary and needs to start with facts and truth, again looking at it from an educator perspective.

The faculty has double responsibilities: to the students—to provide them a sound education that teaches them to be physicians and not just to pass examinations—and to society—which expects graduates to be capable physicians with an ethical and moral foundation comparable to US graduates. In the process of meeting both, we will encounter individuals that are either not motivated or not capable to meet the demands of a medical education. In an effort to reduce the risk of attrition, some schools offer preparatory courses as well as expanded student academic support services to be discussed separately.

Attrition can be induced by the school or by the students.

Schools may have very tolerant admission and performance criteria, and attrition will be low. This likely has an impact on the percentage passing Step 1.

Schools may have high expectations, a very demanding faculty, and difficult internal examinations. This approach leads to high attrition in the first two years and, often, high Step 1 passing rates.

Explanation for such attritions is an imbalance between admission tolerance and academic expectations.

What are some other important factors in causing attrition?

There are students who have no avocation for a career in medicine and are there under pressure from the family. (After all, every family should have a doctor!)

There is a group of students, mainly those recent college graduates, that have difficulties to move from the undergraduate mindset to study the night before a test to the medical school mindset of needing to study every day. Special programs have been developed to change their study habits and may help many and avoid attrition.

There is a group that has been away from college for several years that needs support to revive their study habits. They have the skills and the desire, but they need to be taught how to be in school again. Review and preparation courses before the start of medical school help these students.

There are students who have personal or family issues that distract from their studying. Counseling and support, often available through the school, may help. The problem is having students accept their need of help before they get in academic trouble.

There is another group that did not emphasize the sciences in their undergraduate studies and have problems with courses such as biochemistry or physiology and need support to overcome the problem. Some students have come from a very exact science background, not used to memorize and have problems with some subjects.

There are students whose academic background, based on GPA or MCAT, is mediocre. Stricter admission criteria should have addressed the issue.

Some believe that attrition can be diminished by lowering standards. Well, Step 1 and 2 will cause a lot of disappointment in those students who passed school courses but cannot succeed in the licensing examinations.

Some believe that attrition can be diminished by allowing students to repeat several times one or multiple courses. In these cases we would need data to evaluate their Step 1 and 2 data. But we could anticipate that their competitiveness for residency would be markedly decreased since program directors pay attention to these details, and it is unlikely that they will recruit students with one or more failures in basic science courses.

Attrition is a major problem for students, and it does not good look for the school reputation. It raises eyebrows from regulators and accrediting bodies. Good Caribbean schools are fully cognizant of the attrition issue and are also reminded by the accrediting bodies. It is a challenge to balance the mission to provide students a second chance and an appropriate level of attrition that should be accepted. Once again, schools have a social responsibility toward students who get second chances as well as to society at large in graduating qualified students. The preparatory courses mentioned hopefully address these issues.

Graduation Rate

Graduation rate and attrition rate are major parameters evaluating an academic institution. Graduation rate is determined by how many students complete the course of study in the prescribed period of time. In US medical schools, it has been traditional that students graduate at the end of four years, although now is changing to five or six years. The same could be expected in Caribbean schools.

What is the available information for Caribbean schools? Information is very scanty, hard to obtain, and very difficult to verify.

The information that we could find indicated a 70% graduation rate and a 4 year graduation rate of 60%. This information is in fact incomplete. We need to add to this how many pass Step 1 and 2 and then how many obtain a residency. As an example: If at one school we see an entering class of 200, that means that 140 will graduate (60%). The number that can be expected to match according to the NRMP is 56%—that is 82 of the 140 that graduated. That means that of an initial cohort of 200 entering, only 82 (or 41%) will graduate and obtain a residency. The rest will either have dropped out or will be coming from behind, lowering their prospects of obtaining a residency. This is a theoretical number but likely to be realistic based on published data. That is an abysmal number, especially if we consider that these students will have a debt of almost $200,000 or more.

We will discuss this topic in greater details in a subsequent chapter.

CHAPTER 8

Accreditation of Offshore Caribbean Schools

> Accreditation is the act of granting credit or recognition, especially to an educational institution that maintains suitable standards. Accreditation is necessary to any person or institution in education that needs to prove that they meet a general standard of quality.
>
> —www.vocabulary.com/dictionary/**accreditation**

ACCREDITATION OF UNIVERSITIES and colleges is critically important to guarantee the consumers, students, families, and those financing the education that the institutions meet standards adopted by oversight organizations. These organizations define minimum standards in all areas associated to a teaching institution, curriculum, evaluations of performance, facilities, organization and management, etc. US medical schools, public or private, are accredited by a single agency, the Licensing Commission of Medical Education (LCME). They are responsible to conduct exhaustive visit on periodic basis.

All Caribbean medical schools should have to go through a similar process, preferably conducted by a single organization that evaluates all schools. This would guarantee that all schools operating in the Caribbean meet the same standards. This is extremely important for US students and for the US government that either thru federally funded financial aid, the Veterans Administration or other public organizations help fund student education. I believe that this should be the ultimate goal, a single agency using the same standards conducting accreditation visits to all that receive, directly or indirectly, US funds.

Unfortunately this is not the case. The US Department of Education has not dealt with a single agency that reviews and accredits Caribbean medical schools. It approves national agencies, many created by a local government that appoints an organization that in turn inspects and accredits a medical school. Fortunately, in recent years organizations have been created that accredit colleges and universities in Caribbean countries. Otherwise the accreditation process is determined for each country through a locally appointed board.

I will discuss these issues in some detail. It will be shown that several schools meet standards that are very similar or equal to those that govern the accreditation of US medical schools and some of the accrediting bodies to be described have followed the principles and guidelines of LCME.

At last count more than thirty medical schools have opened or operate in the Caribbean. Some have been around for many years, and a number of them have appeared in the last decade. Some proudly recognize their accreditation by established bodies in the Caribbean. Others simply state that they are listed in some accepted list without explaining by whom and how they receive accreditation. One of the major problems with Caribbean Schools is the lack of a uniform and standardized accreditation process.

In time there will be solutions. As indicated by the ECFMG, and described later, only graduates who have attended schools that have been accredited meeting standards compatible with US standards will be issued a certificate that will allow them to enter postgraduate training. These regulations will go in effect in 2023. Many Caribbean schools will be facing a serious dilemma of investing to make changes to secure accreditation or lose their ability to recruit students planning to practice in the US

Before we discuss accreditation in some detail, let's mention how those schools start.

1) The first step is that the school owners negotiate with the government of an independent country in the Caribbean and obtain an act of the legislature or the government, granting

permission to establish a university or a medical school. The local government must recognize and authorize the school to grant MD degrees. The agreement also outlines advantages and concessions to the new school that will be discussed later, such tax advantages, land utilization, etc.

2) The country then creates an accrediting agency or agree to delegate accreditation to an existing organization. They will evaluate the new school and determine if they meet certain standards.
3) Having completed these steps, the school will be recognized by the country and start operating. At this time it can appear on any lists such as the World Directory of Medical Schools (WDOMS), which was created by merging the IMED from the ECFMG and Avicenna (WHO) directories.
4) If the school wants its students to be eligible for US federal student aid, the agency designated to accredit the school should be reviewed and recognized by an agency of the US Department of Education.

As we mentioned earlier, the accreditation process is variable. Accrediting bodies might be country specific or regional.

Accrediting bodies that are country specific may have little frame of reference to evaluate a medical school. In small islands it is difficult to prove the complete independence of its members and lack of conflict of interest between board members and the school. If US standards are applied, these conflicts of interests or at least the appearance of conflict of interest abound. Some schools have offered a number of advantages to the members of the board not compatible with standard practices in the United States to avoid conflicts of interest.

Some accrediting bodies provide accreditation to several schools in several countries. These accrediting bodies follow guidelines established by the Liaison Committee on Medical Education (LCME), which accredits schools in the United States and Canada.

Accrediting Bodies That Review Schools in a Single Country

- Dominica Medical Board – Accredits Ross University in Dominica.
- Grenada Ministry of Health, Social Security, the Environment, and Ecclesiastical Relations – Accredits Saint George's University in Grenada.
- National Council of Higher Education, Science, and Technology – Accredits several regional medical schools in the Dominican Republic.

It is my opinion that single-country accreditation agencies should be avoided, especially in small countries with small population and not an abundant number of individuals with the knowledge and skills to conduct an accurate and critical inspection.

Multicountry Accrediting Agencies

CAAM-HP

Some time ago some Caribbean countries recognized the need to provide a process that could examine the quality standards of Caribbean schools and universities. This eventually resulted in the creating of CAAM-HP , the Caribbean Accreditation Authority for Education in Medicine and other Health Professions (CAAM-HP)

CAAM-HP was established in 2003 under the aegis of the Caribbean Community (CARICOM) to ensure that the educational programs of medicine and other health professions offered by institutions in CARICOM countries meet international standards. Through its accreditation process, the CAAM-HP provides assurance to students, graduates, the health professions, healthcare institutions, and the public that programs leading to qualifications in medicine, dentistry, veterinary medicine, nursing, and other health professions meet appropriate national and international standards for educational quality, and that the graduates have a sufficiently complete and valid educational experience.

CAAM-HP is an agency of CARICOM. CARICOM is a market union for countries in the Caribbean including Anguilla, Antigua and Barbuda, the Bahamas, Barbados, Belize, Cayman Islands, Dominica, Grenada, Guyana, Haiti, Jamaica, Montserrat, Saint Kitts and Nevis, Saint Lucia, Saint Vincent and the Grenadines, Suriname, Trinidad and Tobago, British Virgin Islands, and Turks and Caicos Islands.

Typically, CARICOM-HP reviews a school or program on a six-year cycle, but they may determine that an earlier review is necessary. A CAAM visit usually includes its members plus guests, often members of US schools with experience in accreditation. Initially, CAAM-HP gives provisional accreditation, and subsequently following a formal site visit, it may give formal accreditation or revoke the provisional accreditation.

CAAM-HP serves as the policy maker and accrediting agency, and its membership is composed of persons nominated jointly by academic institutions in the community offering training in medicine, dental medicine, and veterinary medicine, as well as representatives of civil societies and student, a total of fifteen members.

CAAM-HP has been reviewed and approved by the US Department of Education through the National Committee on Foreign Medical Education and Accreditation (NCFMEA).

Accreditation Commission on Colleges of Medicine (ACCM)

This organization was founded in 1995 by Professor Conor Ward. It is an independent, not-for-profit organization based in the republic of Ireland. ACCM is invited by governments of Caribbean countries which do not have a national medical accreditation body, to act on their behalf in relation to the inspection and accreditation of specified medical school/s in their country.

ACCM has been reviewed and approved by the US Department of Education through the National Committee on Foreign Medical Education and Accreditation (NCFMEA).

The following schools are accredited through ACCM:

- Saint Maarten—American University of the Caribbean (AUC School of Medicine)
- Saba—Saba University School of Medicine
- Cayman Islands—Saint Matthew's University School of Medicine
- Nevis—Medical University of the Americas
- Saint Kitts—University of Medicine and Health Sciences
- Aruba— Aureus University and Xavier University

An important step in the accreditation of a Caribbean medical school, as far as the United States is concerned, is the approval of these accrediting bodies by the National Committee on Foreign Medical Education and Accreditation (NCFMEA). **NCFMEA itself does not accredit schools but is responsible to determine that the accrediting body in a country uses standard practices and processes comparable to those in the United States.**

The United States Department of Education's National Committee on Foreign Medical Education Accreditation (NCFMEA) has set rigorous standards for medical school accrediting bodies to meet. NCFMEA approval of the body that accredits the schools is essential for students attending these schools to obtain the same federally guaranteed student loans made available to students at US medical schools.

We will describe the NCFMEA process in some detail since it is important to understand what it takes for a Caribbean school eventually to become eligible to receive US financial aid. It is a rigorous process that provides assurance regarding the quality of education.

The process used by the US Department of Education as described by the National Committee on Foreign Medical Education and Accreditation (NCFMEA) for reviewing a foreign country's standards for accreditation of its medical schools involves the following:

1) Submission of an application information with all supporting documents (e.g., copies of statute and regulations, standards, examples of site visits, etc.) in English.

2) This is followed by staff analysis and review of the information and documents. The staff member then prepares an analysis based on the documentation provided by the country and the comparability of the country's standards to those in the United States. A copy of the staff analysis is sent to the country for review and comment.
3) Approximately two weeks before the NCFMEA meeting, the department transmits copies of the staff analysis, supporting documentation, and the country's response to the staff analysis (if any) to the NCFMEA members for their review prior to their meeting.
4) **NCFMEA meeting conducts a public session**. A department staff member presents an overview of the analysis of the country's accreditation standards and processes to the committee members and answers any questions committee members might have. After the staff presentation, any official representatives of the country are given the opportunity to present information and answer any questions posed by committee members.
5) Armed with all this information, **NCFMEA members meet in executive session**, which is open to official representatives of the country but is closed to members of the public. During this executive session, the committee discusses the country's accreditation standards and procedures and then makes a determination as to whether the country's system for accrediting medical schools is comparable to the system used in the United States.
6) The decisions reached by the NCFMEA at its meeting are kept confidential until the US Secretary of Education reviews the decisions and issues official notifications to the countries. After the secretary letters are faxed and mailed to the countries and the US Department of State is advised of the NCFMEA decisions, those decisions are made available to the public.

We describe this process in some detail to demonstrate that is thorough and fair. Having been part of several site visits by accrediting bodies both in the United States and in an offshore school, those accreditation visits demand from the school proper preparation and self-study. In 2015 it is difficult to separate if the accrediting visitors come from the LCME, CAAM-HP, or a state medical education body. For example, a CAAM site visit usually includes its members plus guests. Often, members of US schools with experience in accreditation are also part of the visiting team and participate in the report. Personal experience has taught me that these reports are detailed with very pertinent questions and requests for additional information. The visitors not only review documents but also conduct private sessions with groups of students, faculty, and administration.

As indicated earlier, many Caribbean schools indicate in their marketing material that the school is listed, for example, by the World Health Organization. An important difference that must be emphasized is between "accredited" and "listed" or "recognized."

Accredited indicates that the school has undergone a critical inspection and evaluation provided by members of an outside agency. **Listed** is not the same as accredited and usually implies that the government of a country and a local board have approved the school.

Since 2014, to be internationally recognized as an official medical school, it must be **listed** in the directory in the World Directory of Medical Schools (WDOMS), which was created by merging the IMED from the ECFMG and Avicenna (WHO) directories.

According to the US Educational Commission for Foreign Medical Graduates (ECFMG), only students who obtain degrees from schools listed in the WDOMS directory are eligible to take the USMLE exams and participate in residency matching (NRMP).

It is important to note, however, that WDOMS (or IMED/ Avicenna) **is only a directory and *not* an accreditation.** The only requirement for a school to be on the WDOMS directory is to have a government charter from the country in which the school is located.

As indicated earlier, NCFMEA is not an accrediting agency for a medical school but is the reviewer of the accrediting body that reviews medical schools. Being "listed by NCFMEA" could suggest that the school is accredited by a US organization when it only means that the body that reviews and accredits the school is approved by the NCFMEA. We are enclosing the NCFMEA listed schools.

Table 7-1

American University of Antigua (AUA)
American University of Antigua College of Medicine
American University of the Caribbean (AUC)
Medical University of the Americas (MUA)
Ross University
Saba University
Saint George's University (SGU)
Saint Matthews University (SMU)
University of the West Indies

This is a minority of medical schools operating in the Caribbean.

State Accreditation

In addition, to the accreditation steps mentioned above, many states in the United States require that their state board of medical education conducts an independent review, often with additional members from US schools with expertise in education. These state site visits are important since they will determine what the graduate of a school can do in a specific state.

States like California, New York, and Florida require state approval in order for students to do clinical clerkships in those states during their third or fourth years in medical school. State approval is also important for the recruitment of local residents who will attend a school and eventually establish practice in those states. State approval is as important as an accreditation site visit by one of the accrediting bodies mentioned earlier. State approval requires a site visit comparable to an accreditation site visit. The most important state approval is the **California state approval** since California approval is recognized and accepted by several states.

State approval has implications for the schools, and I will discuss it.

California

California accreditation is required for anyone going to do a clerkship or a rotation, to get a residency, or to get a license to practice in California. In addition, *"California's* Approved List *of International Medical Schools,"* is used by other states including Alaska, Colorado, Indiana, New Mexico, and Tennessee. Graduates of officially California-disapproved schools cannot obtain residencies or licensure.

At present, only five Caribbean medical schools are on the California approved list:

- American University of the Caribbean (AUC)
- Saint George's University (SGU)
- Ross University
- Saba University
- American University of Antigua (AUA)

Graduates can therefore practice in California and the numerous other states that follow the California's list.

Caribbean med schools on the *California's Disapproved List* at the moment, include Spartan Health Sciences University, University of Health Sciences Antigua, and Saint Matthew's University (SMU). Graduates from these schools cannot practice in any of the states that follow California's approved list and disapproved list as stated above.

New York

New York accreditation is needed for students from foreign medical schools to conduct more than twelve weeks of clinical rotations in the state and is also required for graduates to obtain residencies in the state.

Approval by New York is important based on the number of students coming from northeastern states, especially New York and New Jersey.

Kansas

The Kansas State Board of Healing Arts has its own list of approved and disapproved schools. In order to get a license to practice in Kansas, you must be a graduate of an approved school or a school that has not been disapproved and the school must have been in operation for at least fifteen years.

According to the Kansas Board of Healing Arts, the following schools, at the moment, are disapproved:

UTESA (Universidad Tecnológica de Santiago), Santo Domingo in the Dominican Republic (Board Decision 8-14-99)

UNIREMHOS (University of Eugenio María de Hostos), Santo Domingo in the Dominican Republic, closed 1998 (Board Decision 8-14-99)

Saint Matthew's University, British West Indies (Board Decision 10-10-06)

Universidad CETEC, Santo Domingo, Dominican Republic, closed 1984 (Board Decision 10-21-11)

Universidad CIFAS Escuela de Medicina, Santo Domingo, Dominican Republic, closed 1984 (Board Decision 10-21-11)

Universidad Mundial Dominicana Escuela de Medicina (World University), Santo Domingo, Dominican Republic, closed 1991

Spartan Health Sciences University School of Medicine, Vieux Fort, Saint Lucia (Board Decision 10-21-11)

University of Health Sciences Antigua School of Medicine, Saint John's, Antigua and Barbuda (Board Decision 10-21-11)

Universidad Federico Henriquez y Carvajal (UFHEC), Santo Domingo, Dominican Republic, closed 1998 (Board Decision 10-21-11)

Kigezi International School of Medicine; Cambridge, England; and Kabale, Uganda (Board Decision 10-21-11)

Texas

Of the offshore Caribbean med schools, only America University of the Caribbean, Saint George's, and Ross are listed as approved in the state of Texas.

We hope that the above discussion has helped in clarifying several points:

- Since 1970 much has changed in the review of medical education in the Caribbean.
- Formal accrediting bodies that follow LCME guidelines have appeared and help differentiate schools.
- Deans of schools and faculty of US schools have actively participated in the schools' site visit as consultants to any one of the accrediting bodies discussed earlier.

Having participated in several site visits one is keenly aware of the strictness of the review and the requirement that the school act on the reviewers' recommendation. Nothing irritates an accreditor more than if the school does not follow recommendations.

All of the above should increase the credibility of the school and dispel some of the concerns voiced by deans and program directors in the United States.

As discussed above, ACCM, CAAM-HP, California, and New York conduct accreditation visits to several Caribbean schools. We believe that such accreditation provides a measure of external review, defined standards of education, and quality.

The enclosed table lists schools that (as of 2015) have not been reviewed by US NCFMEA, CAAM-HP, ACCM, California, and New York, which we consider the major agencies that not only evaluate quality of education but also allow students to do clerkships in those states and allow graduates to practice in those estates.

Table 7-2

	ACCM	CAAM-HP	NCFMEA	California	New York
American International Medical University (AIMU)	No	No	No	No	No
Atlantic University School of Medicine (AUSOM)	No	No	No	No	No
Aureus University School of Medicine	No	No	No	No	No
Avalon University School of Medicine	No	No	No	No	No
Caribbean Medical University (CMU)	No	No	No	No	No
College of Medicine and Health Sciences	No	No	No	No	No
Georgetown American University	No	No	No	No	No
Saint Martinus University	No	No	No	No	No
Saint James School of Medicine (SJSM)	No	No	No	No	No
Texila American University	No	No	No	No	No
University of Health Sciences Antigua (UHSA)	No	No	No	No	No
University of Health Sciences Antigua (UHSA)	No	No	No	No	No

A number of Caribbean schools are not listed here since, as we mentioned, they are accredited by locally appointed accreditation committees. As we indicated earlier, external accreditation committees have a reputation of being stricter, more independent, and thus, enhance the reputation of the institution. Regional schools are accredited by their own national governments and are not part of our review and do not receive many US students. These are schools in Cuba, Dominican Republic, and Haiti.

From a student applicant perspective, this is a very important point. Where is the school recognized and accredited? That will determine what state of the United States will grant a license to practice medicine, an important point to consider in future planning.

I would like to close this section with some comments. We have reviewed the processes leading to medical school accreditation. The accreditation process should include and be used to evaluate quantifiable outcomes. Let me propose the following:

- Class size does not fluctuate by more than 15% from semester to semester. That would demonstrate stability in educational resources.
- 75% of students **entering school** passing Step 1. Reporting Step 1 scores only for student taking the examination does not take into account attrition.
- Mean Step 1 scores of 200. This would guarantee greater probability of obtaining a residency through the NRMP.
- 75% graduating in six years.
- 90% securing a residency and 85% securing residency through the NRMP.

Mandating accreditation standards containing quantifiable outcomes will add a lot to the existing requirements for accreditation. It will also keep schools already eligible for aid on a path for improvement and make the other schools work hard to achieve these standards since financial aid is one of the great recruiter and the only way for a school to qualify for US financial aid is by obtaining approval by NCFMEA.

The above suggestions are not arbitrary. In a 2010 report by the Government Accounting Office suggested the following:

- A 75% institutional pass rate for access to federal student loans. It was anticipated that only 11% of schools would meet this requirement.
- Collect data on graduation rates.
- Require foreign schools to report aggregate licensing examination pass rates and verify this information independently.

I know that schools will resist this, but students will be well served by stricter policies. To achieve the above will be a challenge for everyone, but it will guarantee student applicants that the school will meet measurable criteria reviewed by an external agency.

Accreditation of Caribbean schools will receive a major push in 2023. The ECFMG has stated that **"effective in 2023, physicians applying for ECFMG Certification will be required to graduate from a medical school that has been appropriately accredited. To satisfy this requirement, the physician's medical school must be accredited through a formal process that uses criteria comparable to those established for US medical schools by the Liaison Committee on Medical Education (LCME) or that uses other globally accepted criteria, such as those put forth by the World Federation for Medical Education (WFME)"** (see appendix 2).

This is a major step forward in guaranteeing the quality of Caribbean education. Implementation of these regulations will necessitate major changes in many of the schools that currently operate in the Caribbean. If they want to continue to operate and attract students from the United States, they will need to make substantial improvements. Finally, it should be noted that the Code of Federal Regulations (CFR 600) defines a number of issues regarding offshore medical schools allowed to receive US financial aid. Compliance with CFR is critical for any activity regulated by the federal government.

Lets hope that when universal accreditation has taken place some of the stigma associated to Caribbean education is erased.

CHAPTER 9

Student Recruitment and Admission
How Caribbean Schools Recruit

MOVING FROM AN LCME school to an offshore proprietary Caribbean school is an interesting experience. In a US school, thousands of students apply, and the faculty accepts a limited number of students. Hundreds or thousands of applicants with very good records, are not selected. The decision is commonly based on the academic record. Obviously being the son or daughter of a large donor, an alumnae, or a faculty member may slightly distort this meritocracy.

US medical schools do not need and rarely advertise. There may be some brochures circulated to students, but as a rule, the applicant seeks the school, and the schools do not marketing and advertising. The number of applicants is several times the number of available positions, particularly in those states with only one medical school. This always leaves thousands of applicants out or on a wait list.

Caribbean medical schools, all of them for profit, have to develop a large applicant pool with publicity and marketing. The dominant reality is that the number admitted for a given semester will be determined by the budgetary needs of the school with the academic record of the applicant varying according to the semester and often being a secondary factor. This is not a pleasant comment but is a reality. Schools may have a bottom line for acceptance but not a fixed criteria.

In offshore schools, the recruitment and selection of students have very different approaches than in US schools. The number of students admitted is often resulting from a combination of academic records of the applicants, as determined by the faculty, and the financial needs of the administration, the latter being the major determinant of class size. The academic record of those accepted fluctuates.

Understanding the development and growth of private medical schools in the Caribbean requires information regarding the number of people considering going to a medical school and the existing number of available entry positions in US medical schools. These two numbers give us an estimate of supply (number of positions available in first-year US medical schools) and demand (the number of students who will try to get acceptance to these schools). That is only an estimate since a number of college students look at their academic record and MCAT score and realize that their probabilities of acceptance are very low and apply directly to Caribbean schools.

The Applicant Pool

According to the AAMC, the number of applicants has increased by 38% in the last ten years, and in the same period the number of available positions has increased by only 22%. The gap between applicants and positions has grown despite the efforts to increase class size by many schools and the opening of several new schools. The chances of being accepted have not changed much for those with very good but not stellar records.

The following table clearly demonstrates the gap and shows the total number of applicants (many of whom are likely to have applied more than once) and the number of accepted students. The sources for this information are reports from the Association of American Medical Colleges.

Table 8-1

Year	Applicants	Enrollment	Diff	% Enrolled
2004	35735	16648	19087	53.41
2005	37372	17003	20369	54.50
2006	39108	17361	21747	55.60
2007	42315	17759	24556	58.03

2008	42231	18026	24205	42.68
2009	42268	18390	23878	43.56
2010	42741	18665	24076	56.32
2011	43919	19230	24689	56.21
2012	45266	19715	25551	56.44
2013	48014	20055	27959	58.23
2014	49480	20343	29137	58.88

The increase in the total number of applicants is impressive. Between 2004 and 2014, the number of applicants has increased by 49%. In the same period, the number of *first-time* applicants has increased by 34%.

Who Is Likely to Apply to a Caribbean School?

There will be exceptions but the student with a very high college GPA and very high Medical College Admission Test (MCAT) is not the likely to be an applicant to a Caribbean school. There will be exceptions, but the above will be the general rule.

Looking at number of students considering entry to medical school classified by MCAT score and college GPA will give a better idea of who is likely to be the Caribbean school applicant. In addition to this data, we need to also consider the schools that do not require MCAT as an admission requirement. Unfortunately such a group continues to exist, and many have maintained the "no MCAT" policy and recruit at a different academic level.

The following chart shows the number of students that were rejected by US schools listed by GPA and MCAT. It should give us an idea of the potential pool of applicants to offshore schools.

Table 8-1

GPA	MCAT	Not Accepted	GPA	MCAT	Not Accepted
3.8–4.0	**39–45**	1	**3.0–3.19**	**39–45**	2
	36–35	2		36–38	7

	33–35	17		33–35	31
	30–31	34		30–31	75
	27–29	72		27–29	140
	24–26	89		24–26	340
	21–23	175		21–23	420
	18–20	83		18–20	290
	15–17	46		15–17	224
3.6.3.79	**39–45**	2	**2.8–2.9**	**39–45**	0
	36–38	3		36–35	0
	33–35	32		33–35	9
	30–31	71		30–31	63
	27–29	121		27–29	106
	24–26	209		24–26	172
	21–23	262		21–23	262
	18–20	239		18–20	245
	15–17	107		15–17	151
3.4–3.59	**39–45**	2	**2.6–2.79**	**39–45**	1
	36–35	3		36–35	2
	33–35	32		33–35	11
	30–31	82		30–31	19
	27–29	201		27–29	62
	24–26	313		24–26	128
	21–23	408		21–23	169
	18–20	328		18–20	137
	15–17	171		15–17	106
3.2–3.39	**39–45**	1	**2.4–2.59**	**39–45**	0
	36–35	7		36–35	0
	33–35	30		33–35	0
	30–31	97		30–31	19
	27–29	235		27–29	21
	24–26	338		24–26	51
	21–23	450		21–23	84
	18–20	349		18–20	53
	15–17	205		15–17	66

The total number of applicants not accepted by US medical schools is 7958. A close look at this chart shows 352 applicants with MCAT above 30 and GPAs above 3.4. Unless there were some nonacademic reasons (drug use, criminal record, personality disorders, etc.) these students would instantly be accepted in a Caribbean school!

This chart suggests that many of the 7,598 applicants that were not accepted are potential recruits for offshore schools. This does not count an unknown number who, having lower scores on the MCAT or have noncompetitive GPAs, decide to bypass applying to US schools and go directly the route of offshore schools.

These numbers start to define the pool of potential applicants that will be the focus of attention by Caribbean schools recruiting staff.

What Are the Admission Requirements for Caribbean Schools?

The following are some general principles, and obviously, these requirements will vary from school to school:

- Caribbean medical schools do not have a uniform admission policy, and in many cases, the lower limit of MCAT and GPA for acceptance is determined by the size of the class to be recruited.
- Some schools, not many, have a limit of MCAT or GPA below which they will not consider an applicant or will suggest that they take a preparatory course (more about that later).
- Some schools do not require MCAT—usually the newer schools or those with lower standards. As a school's applicant pool increases, they may become more selective, and that is when they are likely to demand MCAT scores.
- Some look at the personal interview, the MCAT and GPA score, the individual's experience in health professions, personal experiences, and careers prior to applying to medical school. Based on the above, the individual interviewer will make the recommendation, and the faculty admissions committee decide. A good personal interview by an experienced interviewer

allows a more accurate picture of the applicants and perhaps an explanation of reasons for lower MCAT or GPA.

One unfortunate reality is that in many schools, there is no clear differentiation between the interviewer and the recruiter. On the one hand, the person doing the interview is assessing the applicants record, past experiences, personality, and other important factors ., in order to make a recommendation. On the other hand, the individual wearing his recruiter role is trying to explain the wonders of his school and how it is better than the competition. This is a gray area that has not received much attention by accrediting agencies. In my opinion there should be clear demarcation between the recruiter and the interviewer to improve the selection process.

Regardless of the criteria used, the Department of Education requires that admission be a faculty decision made by a faculty admission committee. The decision to admit, in reality, is often made by the faculty but influenced by the administration, which knows how many students need to be admitted to meet their financial needs. As a result faculty and administration often have conflicts, and faculty sometimes may develop a more permissive approach to academic standards. Obviously, this issue could be eliminated if the accrediting entities determine the maximum number of students that a school can admit per class and also a threshold of academic record of applicants.

Admission Requirements, Pros and Cons

On average, enrollees to Caribbean schools have lower GPAs or MCATs than US enrollees. It is at this junction that academic decisions and business decisions may conflict. What are some of the issues?

Is MCAT an Important Predictor of Academic Performance?

Schools that do not require MCAT scores will try to explain that MCAT is not a predictor of performance, especially for minority students. This issue has been previously demonstrated and reported.

Can these conclusions be translated to the pool of applicants-at-large and applicants to Caribbean schools in particular?

Low MCAT score may also be the consequence of students having only a modest command of the English language, having difficulties understanding well the questions or taking too long to answer and not finishing the test.

There is another side to the argument. MCAT has some correlation with medical school performance, but an MCAT score below those reported for students admitted to US medical schools do not indicate a high likelihood of failure. I have seen many students with MCATs ranging from 22 to 20 that, that with proper preparation, especially a preparatory course, do very well in school and pass with very good scores all licensing examination.

MCAT is an important test for medical school admission, and the following are important concepts:

- A report published in *Academic Medicine* (volume 10, 2005) indicated that medical school grades were best predicted by a combination of MCAT scores and undergraduate GPAs, with MCAT scores providing a substantial increment over GPAs.
- MCAT scores were better predictors of USMLE Step scores than GPAs, and the combination did a little better than MCAT scores alone.
- The probability of experiencing academic difficulty tended to vary with MCAT scores.
- MCAT scores were strong predictors of scores for all three USMLE Step examinations, particularly Step 1.

The value of MCAT scores needs to be viewed also from a different perspective. MCAT scores commonly applied by US schools leave out many students who, as demonstrated by the experience of offshore schools, will eventually perform well in the multiple licensing examinations and successfully graduate. On the other hand, students with MCAT scores below 19 indicate, in my experience, a higher risk of academic failure. Indeed, I have seen some exceptions, especially among those with little science background or coming from another career.

From a business perspective, class size determines the financial success of the enterprise and academic standards are often variable. Enrollment will increase by lowering MCAT criteria or not considering MCAT as some schools do! Admitting students with very poor academic records will be followed by high attrition and leave high debts. That is an ethical dilemma to be considered by all Caribbean schools.

This is one of the frequent and often valid criticisms of offshore schools: for financial reasons they will admit a large number of students with low academic credentials and will put them at a high risk of not completing school, not passing licensing examinations, or failing to obtain a postgraduate position. Fortunately several schools, mainly the best known ones, have recognized that and have implemented programs to help students with poor academic records and high avocation for medicine.

Is GPA an Accurate Predictor of Medical School Performance?

A few comments about GPA and Caribbean medical school as criteria for admission. Many factors make comparison of GPAs difficult.

- The GPA is influenced by the college, its type, its reputation, and the ranking of the school. Some schools are more rigorous, and hence, GPAs may be lower. A good example, Canadian schools are more rigorous than US schools, and the result is that few Canadian students ever fail in Caribbean medical schools.
- The GPA is often influenced by the courses taken by the student. Fine arts may improve your GPA, but the truth be known, good schools will calculate science and grades in required courses as a separate GPA score.
- GPAs calculated with a transcript from different colleges represents a problem. Are GPAs from different schools comparable? Why did the student transfer?

- Also, a more recent event is the student who, for financial reasons, will attend a community college and then transfer to a four-year institution. Can the GPA from a community college compare to a highly regarded undergraduate institution?
- Many students who apply to Caribbean schools have completed their college education several years before and are changing careers. How relevant is a GPA if the gap between graduation is of several years?
- What was the major, and how applicable is to the medical school curriculum?
- What year did the applicant complete the science prerequisites? If a long time has passed, are those grades useful?

Analysis and comparison of GPAs become complicated because of the multiple variables mentioned above and many others.

Perhaps performance on required science courses provide a more standardized information.

Some Practices Used by Some Caribbean Schools.

- Accepting students with MCAT of 17 or 15 defines a student at a much higher risk of failing. This could be tolerated if the students are counseled before entering school and they understand the financial risk.
- Requiring or mandating a medical sciences preparatory course could decrease the risks and improve the student chances (more on this later).
- Not requiring MCAT implies that the school is looking at a pool of higher-risk students. In my opinion those who do not ask for MCAT scores will give you a rationalization, not an explanation based on serious evidence.
- Accepting a student with very poor academic records is a high risk for a student who will have to repay all the loans for what there is no forgiveness. His or her acceptance poses an ethical dilemma.

- Admission to medical schools should be limited to those considered to have good chance of graduation. There is plenty of data available to make these predictions, although we know there will be exceptions. As indicated earlier, there is some correlation between MCAT and Step 1 and 2 scores. A very low MCAT should flag risks.
- More important, however, is allowing students with very low GPA. They are likely to be those with very low Step 1 and 2 scores and unlikely to secure a residency position through or outside the match. There are some ethical implications that schools should consider.
- Some of the practices stretch the ethical boundaries of greed and commercialism.

We will discuss later the characteristics of the student body. Many have had other careers that delayed their application to medical school.

Critics of Caribbean school admission practices support the argument that admission of high-risk students is not justified and is only driven by money. Perhaps they should listen to the more than 20,000 graduates currently licensed and practicing in the United States and Canada who were not accepted by US medical schools and were given second chances by offshore schools.

Indeed this is a complicated issue. Caribbean schools very often take many students with low academic records, and this must be accepted as a real risk. Two things are essential, that the student understand the risk and not be given false expectations and that the school give the student the necessary tools to minimize the risk. Also, schools have enough information to predict the student's risk of not graduating and the ethical attitude ought to be advising the student of the risks or simply not admitting. Ethics and business should go together.

Because of the diversity of the applicant pool, the diverse academic performance, different time periods since completing college, and the large number of first-generation Americans with English as a second language, several schools have instituted a twelve- to sixteen-week introduction program that is intense and focused on introduction to medical school courses, reviews of science courses applicable to medical school, learning how to study, and developing good studying habits. These courses are demanding, in some cases with only a 50% pass rate. If a student completes the course successfully, they are guaranteed admission to a Caribbean medical school. These courses have been very successful, and giving the student-at-risk an opportunity to improve the chances of success in the early medical school courses. They will be discussed in greater detail in subsequent chapter.

There only few ways that can allow Caribbean medical schools to continue to grow in numbers or expand the size of their incoming classes.

- Increase the size of the applicant pool through more aggressive marketing. Unfortunately marketing presentations are not necessarily accompanied by supporting accurate data as far as performance, graduation rates and postgraduate success.
- Identifying new group of individuals as potential candidates.
- Lower admission standards. This automatically will increase the potential failure rate.

The issue of class size is often brought up by critics of Caribbean education. This can be a real issue depending on both classroom size and faculty- student ratio and how the curriculum is organized. We will discuss some of these issues in subsequent sections.

The marketing efforts are easy to comprehend and to accept in a competitive world. The changing standards from semester to semester, to meet financial goals, are difficult to understand and even more difficult to justify. When we observe that a school's incoming class size changes from semester to semester without the proportionate increase or adjustments in resources, we have to wonder about the driving forces. Is it business or education? Is it possible to adjust a critical measurement such as faculty-student ratio and quickly ramp up for a large semester? This is an important point that deserves attention and will be discussed at a greater length in a section related to faculty.

CHAPTER 10

A Profile of Caribbean Students

MEDICAL STUDENTS IN a Caribbean medical school are not the cookie-cutter version and what they usually have is their diversity in life experiences, ethnical and cultural backgrounds, age, etc. They all have in common a desire to complete a medical education. Most of them have tried one or more time to enter a US medical school and could not get accepted mainly because of their noncompetitive academic record for US medical school standards. Others thought they were too old, or they were pressured by family.

Applicants to Caribbean medical schools had the determination to go to medical school, They saw in a Caribbean medical school the last opportunity to achieve their goal. A Caribbean medical school was their second and last chance to achieve that dream. Unfortunately, a good number will fail, either because they do not have the necessary academic record, dedication, commitment, or capabilities.

For many, dedication and concentration and the support of dedicated faculty help them succeed. They are the ones whom all the negative reports about Caribbean schools do not talk about. They will graduate and start residency training and will be thankful with the opportunity they were given. For the other group, they failed for any of multiple reasons—they decided to attend medical school without true avocation, attended school often because of social or family pressures, or had a faulty perception of their qualifications or capabilities. There are many reasons why students fail and we will mention them as we proceed.

The demographic of Caribbean student population is very similar to students at US schools.

Table 9-1

	US Schools		Caribbean School	
	Male	Female	Male	Female
White Non-Hispanic	58.12	52.25	60.1	58.75
Asian	19.58	21.28	19.3	19.79
Black Non-Hispanics	4.5	7.97	4.9	4.78
Hispanics	4.03	4.06	4.2	3.59

The following are the demographic averages of students entering Caribbean medical school:

- Age is almost equally divided, 50% of students are 29 or under, and the remaining 25 or under with a very small percentage under 21. The youngest student I have seen was 19 years old (he graduated) and the oldest was 57 years old on admission (he did not graduate).
- 80% are either US citizens or permanent residents and the remaining are either Canadians (10%) or of multiple other nationalities. The number of Canadian students is increasing since schools are making an effort to market themselves in Canada and in addition, the demand for admission to Canadian schools greatly exceeds the capacity of schools.
- The gender proportions vary slightly from semester to semester, but on average is 54% males and 46% females.
- Students are recruited from all over the United States. Several years ago those from New York and New Jersey constituted the majority. In the last few years, the number of students from the West Coast or from Florida has increased substantially, but they come from everywhere in the United States. I had one student from Guam—multiple long flights at the end of every semester!
- The average academic record for the more prestigious schools in the Caribbean is
    - MCAT: 24
    - GPA: 3.2

- Science GPA: 3.1

Other schools have much lower criteria. Some do not require an MCAT score and some do not require an undergraduate degree but a number of credit hours in a college!

In the many years that I met, taught, or interviewed Caribbean students, I internally subdivided them into several groups. My thought never got into the official evaluation.

The first group is "**How come you did not get accepted into a US school?**" They are the proof that admission criteria can miss very good people and class sizes are too small. They had all the qualifications but somehow did not make the cut. Why is that they did not make it? Perhaps they had a bad interview or perhaps a bad interviewer. This process is not an exact science, and many imponderables come into play. They will be the stars of the school, and you do not have to worry about them. I will never understand the reasons. Maybe the interview did not go well, or there were too any applicants better than them—who knows!

A second group is composed of students **with almost competitive MCAT and GPA**. They are the bottom of US admission lists and often wait-listed. They will do OK and complete school with excellent records. They represent the silent majority, never in academic or personal difficulties and perhaps the shining stars of their class.

The third group represents the largest number of students: **"If you work hard and study hard, we will help you make it."** Admission to US schools is heavily determined by MCAT scores or GPA, and the student has to be outstanding to make the cut. Caribbean students often did not have a competitive GPA, either because they got distracted in the early years of college (a son of a friend once said, "In my freshman year, my social life interfered with school") or because for economic reasons they had to work full-time to complete college. Another reason is that their MCAT scores were low, often because poor preparation or knowledge deficiencies in the sciences. They may have major language difficulties or English as a second language. Some of them have a great academic record but have been away from school in other careers for years. These people, if they work hard and school provides them a pre-admission preparation as well as tutoring, will have a good chance of doing well.

A fourth group is composed of **second-career applicants**. These students, several years away from college, had a successful work career, often in health care (nurses, pharmacists, emergency technicians, radiology technicians, military corpsman). They decided that medicine was their field and will work at becoming a physician. They come to school with practical and clinical foundations but lack the basic science education. They often know what it is wrong and how to treat, but they do not know the why, the physiologic and pathophysiological mechanism. Their motivation is high, and they do quite well. They are usually serious and dedicated.

A fifth group, **the older students**. They are of all ages and have seen people in their fifties start medical school. They should be admired but often develop academic difficulties. This is usually a small group of people in their forties or fifties. They always had the dream of becoming a physician. Multiple reasons directed many of them to a different professions or occupations. Many come from previous careers in IT, engineers, teachers, lawyers, investment bankers, etc. They have the money and decided to try. Their success is variable.

Finally there is always a group of **"I do not know what you are doing here"** and occasionally **"Who admitted you?" Your record is very weak, and it will be a struggle. Your GPA and MCAT are low and I do not know why they admitted you**. Your chance of failing is very high. Use all the academic support you can get, and you may have a fighting chance. Was anyone in the admission process able to detect that?

The best way to illustrate the students at Caribbean schools is to present some brief stories of real students we worked with. I would like to describe several cases that illustrate the diversity of a Caribbean school student body and what a second chance can do if given to those that you estimate have potential. They all have graduated and completed their residencies and are now in practice.

These are factual stories of students I knew and followed during my years with the school.

- **CM** is currently a family practitioner in western North Carolina. He served in the US Army as a medic and saw combat with Special Forces. After discharge he thought of going to school and becoming a nurse or physician assistant. Influenced by advertising, he decided to apply to a Caribbean school and completed his education in the prescribed time. After a family practice residency, he returned to his native North Carolina and established a family practice office as well as a clinic to serve lower-income families in the area. He joined the North Carolina National Guard and completed a deployment to Afghanistan.
- **DM** was born in Cuba. He escaped communism, migrating to the United States where he worked as a hospital assistant while completing college. He enrolled in a Caribbean school and graduated from after recovering from very serious illness requiring a bone marrow transplant. He completed an internal medicine residency and is now a hospitalist in Ohio. Few people I know have suffered so many setbacks in life as he did. He was determined to complete his medical education despite financial, personal, and health problems He should serve as a role model to all, and we are very proud of him.
- ***MH** was born and raised in the Washington area and the son of a physician. He spent several years working as an emergency room technician and a cardiology technician. Not accepted in US schools, he entered a Caribbean university. Graduating one year ago, he is currently doing an emergency medicine residency in the Southwest. With a keen love for cardiovascular medicine and personal work experience, he devoted many hours teaching other medical students the basics of clinical cardiology.
- ***MJ** was a young, very intelligent, gregarious individual when she entered medical school. Those of us who met her noticed the intellectual potential but recognized that she needed to grow up. She passed courses, but she also failed a couple that her placed at risk for academic dismissal. She managed to get herself in situational trouble but was never responsible of causing the trouble. Some of us were not willing to see her natural talents go

to waste and some wanted her dismissed from school. A group of senior professors and counselors overruled the others and gave her a chance. The happy end of the story is that today she is a successful practicing surgeon in a Southeastern metropolitan area. People like MJ is what make us believe that people have potential that may not be recognized by simple academic records without a careful examination of the whole person.

- ***RK** came to the school as a basic science professor having completed his PhD at an excellent university. He excelled at his teaching and his creativity and then decided to go to medical school. He entered school, and as expected, he traversed with a great record. After completing his surgical residency, he is finishing a fellowship in colorectal surgery at a major academic center.
- ***JL**'s premedical school career would surprise everyone. He completed college and dedicated himself to jet skiing, becoming a professional jet ski racer and then came to medical school! He completed school with an excellent record and concurrently finished his MBA via distance education. After an emergency medicine residency, he is now practicing in the Midwest.

These are just a few examples observed when I was dean. We could write about hundreds who now are not only successful practitioners but have also excelled in multiple administrative positions both in civilian as well as military life. The above examples identify some characteristics common to the good student in a Caribbean school. They know that for whatever reasons, they were not selected by a US medical school. Their motivation and dedication directed them to an offshore school, the only way they could achieve their dream of one day becoming a physician. They endured the limitations in comfort of a developing country, the weather, the bugs, the lack of entertainment they had in the United States, but they had the desire, motivation, and resiliency to achieve their goal. They have true grit!

These are the ones who make us proud of having played a role in their development, and we are proud of their success.

There is also a small group that you try not to remember but that we have to recognize. You will never understand why they came to medical school and rapidly accumulate enough failures to be eligible for dismissal. The process of dismissal is that they file an appeal to a faculty committee that makes a recommendation to the dean. Some few cases have real-life crises that destroyed their ability to study and could be allowed to repeat. An then there is the other group. The stories they can create are enough for several soap operas. How many relatives can die in a sixteen-week period? How many parents or grandparents in a family are diagnosed with cancer in one sixteen-week period? The decision is obvious—for whatever reason, they will not make it medical school and should be dismissed. One needs to keep in mind one's responsibility to society at large.

The life of a medical student is hard everywhere but specially in many of the Caribbean islands. In either place, the United States or the Caribbean, studying medicine is a full-time occupation. In the United States there are many distractions: movies, theaters, shopping, family, and even dangers such as recreational drugs, but thep to entertain you and cope. We do not want to talk about drugs, but we know they are there and everywhere.

In the Caribbean, the choices are more limited. If you are athletic and a sportsman, the outdoor is great—hiking, canoeing, beach, etc. In the absence of shopping, movies, theaters, and family, these are the activities that make a student's life enjoyable, and many will remember them. But there are also those who do too much of the wrong thing. Drinking or drugs become the escape mechanism and often lead them to academic difficulties.

A Caribbean student needs to maintain contact with family and friends as a support system. The cell phone is always present. A constant sight it is a student walking around with a cell phone. But there is hope, and in a few months, they start their clinical training and are back in the United States. "Off the rock" as they usually describe it.

Drugs are an issue, but I do not have statistics to compare drug use between US students and Caribbean students. Situational depression enhanced by the environment, the loneliness, and the demands from school are a reality, and it keeps the counselors busy. The majority of students cope well, but a minority—and especially those not excelling academically—are usually the victims. All are factors that contribute to attrition, a topic discussed.

It is easy to understand the stress in a Caribbean student life. The material to be covered is the same as any US allopathic school, the semesters are shorter, and they commonly have to memorize concepts with little discussion and reasoning. No wonder attrition is higher than US schools.

The innumerable critics see only that the school exists only to extract money from unsuspecting individuals. Those of us who have been involved with a good Caribbean school saw the sacrifices and the efforts that these students make. You see the signs of stress at the time of final examinations. And then you see the massive exodus toward the airport. For two or three weeks, they will be home, eat good food, and have the opportunity to relax and enjoy life. At the end of those few weeks, it's back to the airport and start all over again.

Please do not think that everything is fine. In that student population, you will find the alcoholic, the substance addict—for these counseling might be of help. For the others—the pathological liar, the cheater, the abuser—all you can hope is that the faculty members identify them and put them through the administrative process and prevent them from graduating.

Attending medical school is not a right but a privilege, regardless of race, sex, or religion. A student's behavior from the very beginning must be like the physician he is trying to become. Schools can provide academic assistance but should not allow student to stay on if he cannot perform academically. Allowing them to repeat course after course does not help anyone. It will be difficult for these individuals to secure a residence or pass all licensing examinations, and it does not help the school reputation. The faculty and the school have a responsibility to society, not just to the student.

CHAPTER 11

Faculty

KNOWLEDGE OF THE sciences, necessary to teach in a medical school, is available worldwide. In any medical school, you will find very talented professors with up-to-date knowledge and great teaching skills. The challenge and the secret for Caribbean schools is to find them and successfully recruit them to join the faculty of a proprietary private school in a distant island of the Caribbean, often known for its tourism and often underdeveloped. Recruiting is always a challenge, and those who do it deserve my respect. When done professionally and consistently, it is possible to identify and select individuals who will do an outstanding job.

Obviously, the results of the recruiting will be influenced by the school reputation as well as its willingness to pay competitive salaries. It is not difficult to find below-average faculty who have been changing transferring from Caribbean school to Caribbean school every two years because of a mediocre performance.

Hiring experienced, high-quality faculty is much more difficult and requires dedicated staff. What are some of the issues associated with recruiting faculty for a Caribbean school?

Identifying candidates requires a very wide network that will direct potential candidates to the school. Person-to-person recruiting is often quite helpful. They could be former or current faculty, former students, or staff. Information given to the candidate on an initial conversation should be accurate. All my many years being involved with faculty recruitment, both in the US and the Caribbean, convinced me that an applicant deserves accurate information if you expect the individual to make a major career decision and develop trust in the institution.

Many potential candidates have little knowledge of Caribbean schools. Those doing the recruiting need to explain to a candidate—who often has taught for years at a medical school in the United States, Canada, or another country—about the existence of for-profit medical schools in the Caribbean. The recruiter must present to the potential candidate accurate information about the school if you want to convince the individual about the seriousness of the institution.

Experience has taught all of those who have worked in a Caribbean school that everywhere in the world there will individuals, regardless of nationality, who run into difficulties and look at a Caribbean school as a place to hide their past and hope that no one will dig deeply and give them a job. In all these years, we have encountered people who have lost their medical license for a multiplicity of reasons—people who had mental health issues that rendered them unfit to be members of a faculty, drug addiction, criminal records, family issues; people who are running away to not pay alimony or away from court injunctions; and many other reasons. Interview and selection ought to be careful and deliberate.

Schools cannot and should not hire faculty who are running away from home because their license was suspended or revoked or they have serious personal issues since it will have a negative impact in the reputation of the school.

A visit to the school is essential. As opposed to the common practice for most positions in US schools, for Caribbean schools, you are recruiting a family, and it is important that the family unit feels comfortable with the environment, the island, and its facilities. Most candidates have already thought and discussed a move to the Caribbean, but what they need from a visit is to learn the details of the job and, above all, learn the practical issues of daily life. Because, yes, the Caribbean may look to most like paradise, but there are many items and services not available in this paradise. If the school is looking for a long commitment, it is essential that the whole family accepts where they are considering the move. Not all Caribbean islands are the same, and the degree of economic development and material things are not available everywhere. Some recruitment failed because the spouse could not become comfortable with the island and the job opportunities or the school for the children. I remember one who, during the interview, asked how long the opera season was! Big red flag—this is not your place.

Recruiting in the Caribbean is family recruiting. Other faculty needs to participate to make the candidate and family feel welcomed and wanted in largely an expatriate, multinational, multicultural community. That is an important aspect. Since an unhappy family in a foreign country will erode, the likelihood of that faculty member's stay on island several years erodes too.

Yes, working in a Caribbean island can be very attractive, but consider the following:

- Are the candidate and their family able to adapt to the smallness of the island?
- Will the faculty member and family adjust to a quasirural life that could be lacking many things like theaters, shopping malls, great restaurants, etc.? Regardless of how developed the island appears or how active the tourism is, they mostly remain developing countries with limited resources. I remember a candidate that asked me about theater and opera in the island. He could have been a great professor, but he would have been very unhappy lacking these things he considered important
- Is there adequate housing available to meet the family expectations? Someone from the school must spend time showing them around.
- How accessible is travel back to the home country? Some islands have several major airlines connecting to Europe and several major cities in the United States. Some have one or two flights a day to Puerto Rico or another Caribbean island, which can add to the cost and time consumption of travel.

The interviewers must be very candid with the candidate to avoid disappointments and the unhappiness of a new faculty members who could not adjust to reality of the circumstances after they settled in.

Recruiting faculty for a Caribbean school must be done with a true presentation of facts. Each island has its own peculiarities, and the facts need to be presented clearly. The candidate and family must have an organized visit of the island to gain firsthand the reality.

Caribbean medical schools do not have many large faculties. Collegiality then becomes an important factor since faculty will be part of the same social network, essentially an expatriate community The personality of the individual will influence their quality of life and social adaptation. There is little room for real prima donnas or troublemakers. Faculty and spouses need to become involved to asses these aspects of a candidate.

It is expected that the potential faculty member present a lecture or some teaching activity and that can be observed and evaluated by members of the faculty. Preferably, more than one candidate will be interviewed so comparisons and evaluations will be done. Involvement of several faculty members as well as students both in meeting, interviewing, and evaluating candidates is a good idea, Students often can recognize a bad teacher before the faculty will admit to it.

Caribbean schools often are playing catch-up and, as they say in sports, "They do not have a big bench." Positions are available and the school will rarely pass up a very good candidate, but sometimes the school has to accept the B team because someone needs to teach the subjects. If that is the case, the school may be better off with a visiting professor for some lectures than settling with a weak candidate.

If all proceeds well, an offer will be made, and then the school will wait for a decision very often influenced by family, with issues such as housingage of children, health issues of older parents, etc.

Since the teaching in the Caribbean is mainly that of the basic sciences, we will talk about that faculty first. They must have to have the knowledge and skills to teach medical students. They all must have a doctorate degree and good command of the English language. They can be recruited from many countries, and that is essentially the approach taken by all Caribbean schools. Faculty will be recruited from the United States, Canada, England, Scotland, Ireland, Hungary, Africa, Austria, India, Nigeria, South Africa, and many other countries. Many foreign faculties were educated or lived in English-speaking countries, so their command of English is very good. In fact, a good command of English must be a requirement.

We have met and worked with the best, which included former chairs of departments in US or Canadian schools, authors of commonly used textbooks, and tenured faculty from major European schools. They are all looking for the same thing: a second career in a very touristic environment with good weather and good beaches. Students benefitted from the experience of senior faculties because of their experience. They hit the ground running. They know the discipline, had lectured many times before, and little orientation was necessary.

We also met the worst, the lazy, the discontent, and those with bad track records. Vetting failed, and we all have tried to forget them. We all make mistakes.

Basic science faculty can be broadly grouped in three categories:

- Retired Americans or Canadians or Europeans. They are experienced and not yet ready to retire completely. They are attracted by a better climate, the beauty of the Caribbean, and a reasonably stress-free life. They have years of experience, so they enter the system very easily and often with good ideas and suggestions. Many of them have retired from senior positions in excellent Canadian or American schools, having been either professors or department chairs.
- A second group is composed of young postdoctorals, many on their first jobs. Multiple reasons attract them to a Caribbean school, but mainly, they are the type of PhDs who like to teach and have limited interest in a research career. Most US schools are looking for faculty who bring or attract research funds, so those who are inclined to pursue a teaching career are, in the eyes of many, less competitive. A school that concentrates on teaching becomes attractive to a young PhD who decided that a research career is not their goal. Young faculty starting their teaching career in a Caribbean school will acquire in twelve months three years' worth of teaching experience since

most schools have new classes three times a year. This quickly accumulated experience is one of the reasons that most junior PhD educators are able to obtain good jobs in any one of the new US schools and some in older prestigious schools.

- Many schools have heavy reliance on a group that originates from developing countries. Many of them are quite good, but they move abroad for better salaries. These individuals are likely to stay in the Caribbean for a long time since salaries, even in the lowest cases, will remain competitive with their home country, and if they perform well, they will have good job security. Caribbean countries are peaceful and safe, something we cannot say about other parts of the world.
- Another group is difficult to describe. Any medical school has examples. Regardless of age, they talked themselves into being fired from one school and jumped to another that happens to be short of needed faculty. They have created the Caribbean circuit from school to school and rarely to better schools. They will quickly demonstrate that either they cannot teach, have previously undetected skeletons in their closet, or are lazy and thought that a Caribbean medical school was a well-paid vacation in a sunny island. If you are recruiting, stay away from them. They are never at fault, and problems are always the dean's fault. If they taught as much as they complained, they would be the busiest faculty members!

For US candidates the salary becomes attractive once you count the tax advantages, which are real. US tax laws allows, in 2015, the first 100,000 of a citizen's salary working overseas not to be subject to federal income tax. This makes many Caribbean salaries very competitive. As a professor who left for a job in a US school and returned two years later said, "Before I had money and no place to spend it, go back home and have plenty of things to spend money on but do not have not enough money to spend."

For individuals from other nationalities, many of them have made careers as expatriates teaching in medical schools anywhere in the world.

Even if some of the schools do not pay exorbitant salaries, they are higher than what is paid in their own country. Once again, if you have a good selection process, you will find people who will do very well and become highly respected faculty members.

Retention is another issue. Most people who are recruited understand the quality of life issues, the work, and the pluses and minuses of island life. But the question remains as to how invested are they and how long they plan to stay. Contracts are commonly for one year, with a clause that the school will notify the faculty member with six month's notice if the contract will not be renewed (usually because of performance issues). Because the same way, you may bring in an outstanding teacher, a gifted lecturer who creates great bond with students, and you want to keep them forever—you will need to be able to offer multiyear contracts. But you will also run into the lazy one, the difficult one, the drunk, the poor teacher, or the one who has lost his medical license for any of multiple reasons, who has jumped bumped from school to school and has never settled anywhere, managing to conceal the issues. The school needs to create contractual coverage that allows for termination for cause. On this issue you need to be firm. The school reputation is harmed if you either recruit or retain the wrong people.

What are some of the reasons people leave or do not take jobs?

- A few will leave because of family reasons. The spouse does not adjust and wants to go home. That is uncommon. People have made a decision to go to the Caribbean and seek a new lifestyle.
- Sometimes spouses had good careers in their country and tried to work from a distance. Sometimes it works, but sometimes it does not. If the spouse decides to go home, you can expect the faculty member to depart shortly after.
- Some leave after a few years because children have grown and need to change schools, go to high school, start working on college application, etc.
- Some leave because they were recruited to a US medical school. There are two factors that in recent years that enhanced recruitment from Caribbean school's young faculty to US

> schools. The teaching experience of a faculty member in the Caribbean grows very quickly if you have three incoming classes every year, and good new, young educators will take advantage and develop experience quickly. New schools need good educators and not people who want to focus primarily on research.

How many professors does a school need? Obviously it depends on the size of the school. The student-faculty ratio in US schools has been reported to be between 0.6:1 to 7:1. For Caribbean schools, the data is often concealed or not reported, the only data available is 7:1 to 13:1.The student-faculty ratio reported by Caribbean schools is quite comparable for ratios seen in undergraduate education.

The faculty to student data for Caribbean schools needs to be scrutinized. It is easy to play with numbers. Are these numbers given representing only people with direct educational activities involving medical students? We have seen reports that include, as faculty, all expatriates in administrative, nonteaching positions. If that is the case, the number of faculty is exaggerated.

Some schools hire recent graduates who did not match or are waiting for the next match as instructors, even if they do not have any clinical or educational experience and just finished medical school. They function as teaching assistants. In US schools they likely not even be considered interns or PG1 and would not be included as faculty or used to calculate ratios. I have seen, in this category, graduates who could not obtain a residency after two years. Should they be counted as faculty? Should they be retained? Inflated numbers do not help the school reputation and only increases lack of respect in the United States for Caribbean schools.

Finally, the issue of quality teaching needs to be mentioned. This is a very difficult topic, and all schools have outstanding professors and some very bad professors. How to deal with the issue is beyond this topic and is more related to the processes associated with evaluation. Some Caribbean schools have initiated vigorous programs to evaluate quality of teaching, both in the basic sciences and clinical sciences.

This information has allowed adjustments in curriculum as well as evaluations of clinical teaching sites. Over time, schools continue to improve. In fact, evaluations are in many cases more formal and critical than some US schools, and this applies both to basic sciences and clinical sciences.

Faculty retention may become an issue. Some faculty expatriates enjoy the work, the quality of life and may stay for many years, build a house, and become part of the society. Others, will forever be expatriates and live in the isolated world of expatriate faculty. How long they will stay is difficult to predict. In many cases, how long they will stay will be a function of family issues or new job opportunities in the United States.

Faculty teaching clinical sciences are often dispersed since Caribbean schools operate with a system of distributed clinical education, operating multiple sites in the United States and sometimes in England. The multiplicity of hospitals used and the diversity of faculty raises multiple issues that make assuring quality experiences and education across all sties teaching sites a complicated process. Often there was little if any integration in teaching content or quality control. Communication and discussions between basic science faculty and the clinicians occurred infrequently.

Things are changing, especially in those considered the best Caribbean schools. The credentials of clinical faculty are reviewed by a faculty committee of the school and given clinical faculty appointments. Regular evaluations submitted by students are reviewed by department chairs and deans. Those processes are in continuous development and will result in significant selection and improvements. Some schools are evolving from part-time chairs whose responsibility was mainly limited to auditing hospital sites to full-time chairs fulfilling the more classical role of department chairs. All these changes, occurring in the best schools, are part of the growth and maturation of some Caribbean schools that are doing their best to reach a quality level comparable to US schools.

Both, because schools' growth and improvement as well as some changes in regulation and the result of recommendation by accrediting agencies, constructive changes have occurred in many schools in teaching methods, testing and evaluation processes. In brief, progression toward medical schools gradually resembling US schools is taking place. This progress is not universal among Caribbean schools. There are several schools tied to the old model and looking to maintain the status quo and the profit margin. Their faculty, graduation rate, and residency placement reflects both the quality and the reputation.

CHAPTER 12

Caribbean Schools' Approaches to Correct Student Weaknesses Preadmission Review Programs and Special School Curriculum

A NUMBER OF CARIBBEAN applicants do not have the academic background expected to succeed in medical school. Their applications show lower MCAT scores and lower GPAs. Many apply several years after completing courses, and many had to return to school to either improve their GPAs or to complete required science courses. The spectrum of applicants is quite wide, as we discussed in a previous chapter. A substantial number could succeed, but they may be facing the risk of either failing school or failing courses unless they are offered some additional opportunities.

Caribbean schools offer students a second chance. Having interviewed many applicants, it was clear that some students had the avocation and motivation, but they were not prepared to study medical sciences and often lacked the foundation of scientific knowledge required to progress in medical school.

The school understands it, and the student understands it. Everyone must accept that these students are at higher risk of failure resulting in higher attrition rate than US schools. Several Caribbean medical schools have examined this issue, and in an effort to prepare them better for the rigorous experience of a medical school presented at an accelerated pace have created review programs to address these disadvantages.

Different approaches were taken to help these students.

- **Create specialized preadmission courses** to teach how to study better, to review good study methods, and to introduce basic concepts that will be needed in medical school.
- **Create a special curriculum** that slows down the pace of teaching. Traditionally Caribbean schools offers a more accelerated pace for the basic science curriculum, often too fast for many students. The choices were simple for these students, either decrease the amount of material presented (probably increasing failure rate on Step 1), or decrease the pace of instruction. Decreasing content may be difficult since Step 1 may ask questions on topics not covered. The second choice is to slow down the pace of teaching for those who need more time at the very beginning to learn some topics.

  The decision to transfer students to the deaccelerated curriculum must be and is made earlier, often during the first semester. The decision could be made by the students who request transfer or by the school that dictates the need to transfer.
- **Some schools have created specialized centers to help students.** They have dedicated faculty to help students with special needs. Schools have hired faculty, not because of their specific knowledge of a discipline but with the qualifications of special education teachers who concentrate in teaching how to study and how to learn.
- **Enhance support services.** One thing quite common in Caribbean schools is the one-on-one assistance offered by professors. Professors are often available to answer questions during office hours or in an unscheduled time. Also, e-mail has become a frequent tool used by students and quickly responded by the professor.
- **Student tutoring** is another approach offered. Senior students that have obtained excellent grades in a discipline meet with one or a group of students to explain topics and answer questions. They are often compensated by the school.

An additional semesters have been added by many Caribbean schools to introduce students to clinical topics and hospital practices preparing them to enter their clinical years. This will be discussed later.

Preadmission Review Programs

Preparatory instruction prior to entry into medical school has been offered in US universities for many years. There are dozens of postbaccalaureate premedical programs that offer students a chance to take science classes like organic chemistry, molecular biology, physics, etc. These programs are held at schools ranging from lesser-known institutions to prestigious medical institutions like Johns Hopkins University.

Are these programs worth it? Yes, but with several caveats. Medical school admissions counselors and admissions officials say: for students who are struggling through their undergraduate work but still yearn to attend medical school, a postbaccalaureate program is typically the best chance to make an improvement. Enrolling in a master's program in science or a master's in public health are other options, but they take longer and can be more expensive and do not offer guarantee of admission.

Postbaccalaureate programs tied to top-ranked medical schools boast that between 80 to100 % of graduates get accepted into medical, osteopathic, dentistry, or nursing schools. Some schools, have links to medical schools, These alliances may open the door to applicants who have completed these preparatory courses.

The following is a list of schools that offer programs that help students improve the chances of acceptance to medical school.

- Boston University—MA in Medical Sciences
- Drexel University College of Medicine—IMS
- Georgetown University School of Medicine—SMP
- New York Medical College—Basic Medical Sciences
- Temple University SOM—Postbaccalaureate program
- University of Cincinnati COM—Special Masters Program

- Eastern Virginia Medical School—Medical Master's Program
- Tufts University SOM—MBS in Biomedical Sciences
- Duke University SOM—Master of Biomedical Sciences
- Northeastern Ohio Universities COM—MD Partnership
- Mount Sinai SOM—MS in Biomedical Sciences
- Philadelphia College of Osteopathic Medicine—Biomedical Sciences
- Rosalind Franklin University—Master of Science in Applied Physiology
- Tulane University—Cell and Molecular Biology
- University of Texas at Dallas—Postbaccalaureate Program
- University of Maryland (College Park)—Science in the Evening

Some Caribbean schools, such as Ross University, the American University of Antigua, and the University of Health Sciences (Saint Kitts) offer similar preparatory programs that are non-ndegree granting. Descriptions of these programs are offered below, and they exist fundamentally for the following purposes.

- To expand recruitment. Students who successfully complete these programs can enter medical school directly with the next entering class. On occasions, up to fifty new students in a semester started medical school through these programs.
- To improve academic qualifications of applicants. These programs are structured to improve students' learning skills and also introduce them to concepts that will be taught in depth in the medical school curriculum. This should decrease the risk of failure in the earlier semesters.
- Give students who have been away from formal education the opportunity to regain the skills they may have lost over the years and prepare them to go through a very demanding academic program.
- Give students coming from different careers or professions an opportunity to increase knowledge of scientific principles.

- Decrease attrition. Over several years, the record has shown that students who complete these programs do academically well and frequently perform as well as many students that came to school with very good academic records.

These programs offer classes presenting introductory information of material to be taught in medical school courses. These courses do not have the depth of medical school courses but discuss the fundamental principles of the discipline and facilitate future understanding.

- Anatomy
- Histology
- Physiology
- Molecular and cell biology
- Biochemistry
- Microbiology
- Genetics
- Immunology
- Behavioral sciences
- Pharmacology
- Epidemiology
- Ethics and professionalism

Also presented are sessions on how to study and be more successful at learning such as

- active and passive learning,
- understanding multiple-choice questions for exams,
- listening and learning during lectures,
- concept mapping, and
- the basics of medical terminology.

To encourage everyday learning and prepare students for a future rigorous medical school curriculum, these programs regularly give quizzes with USMLE-style multiple-choice questions that test understanding and retention of previously taught concepts.

All these courses are very demanding, and in order to pass, the student needs a score of 70% or better. The failure rate is sometimes as high as 40%. The positive sides are listed below side is that,

- Students passing these courses are offered direct admission to the schools or can apply to any other Caribbean school.
- For those students who fail, it gives them a reality test as to why they were not likely to succeed in medical school. Some withdraw during the course, and some even after the very first quizzes.
- The students who accept admission to the school have developed social and study groups. These groups often continue on the island, providing a helpful social network that assists them in the social adjustment and in the academic success.

Many students who completed these courses and proceeded to graduate were considered the least likely to either be admitted or graduate from medical school. When these students pass Step 1 and Step 2, they prove how inaccurate medical school admission criteria are. Students who initially were rejected or not even considered candidates for medical school in a US school as well as a Caribbean school have successfully completed medical education and have now completed residency and are in practice. That is one of the satisfactions of a teaching career.

CHAPTER 13

Curriculum and Didactic Methods

THE CORE CONTENT of all allopathic medical schools worldwide must have substantial comparability. Medical knowledge transcends frontiers and cultures. All medical schools must teach scientific disciplines that provide the fundamental knowledge for a student to become a physician. Everyone needs to learn anatomy, physiology, microbiology, pharmacology, and other disciplines.

From its origin, Caribbean school curriculum planners implemented a curriculum designed to replicate the curriculum in US medical schools. This had to be done because the majority of students were American citizens who, in time, would return to be licensed in the United States. There was no creativity in curriculum design, but the implementation of the curriculum had to be structured to accommodate content to a semester that was often shorter than that in US schools. The concept of an overall accelerated curriculum became an early marketing tool that tried to compensate for the students living overseas in a developing country.

This approach worked fine for the students who came ready to undertake the medical education that they could not get in the United States. For many, they encountered a system that could easily lead to failure. Weaker students had to learn the same in a shorter time and should have required different teaching approaches that only know are being incorporated.

The teaching methods used in Caribbean schools are similar to US schools, have evolved over the years, and consisted of the following:

Didactic

A) *Lectures.* For many years, lectures represented the main teaching format. They were organized by discipline with little interconnection with other disciplines At present there is a growing tendency to reduce the number of lectures and place more emphasis in small group learning. Lectures, however, remain an essential component of teaching. At present everyone agrees that a lecture is a very passive way to transmit knowledge and information, and new approaches are needed.

B) *Problem-based learning.* It was implemented to promote self-learning and create a method to encourage students to research information and reason through a problem. It was always presented in addition to lectures.

C) *Organ-based system curriculum.* This is the new way of thinking. Disciplines organize their teaching around an organ system. It will work, but still in stages of organization and implementation. It necessitates bringing down discipline walls, controlling faculty egos, and creating a true multidisciplinary planning.

D) *Simulators.* The teaching of basic clinical concepts in the Caribbean is often limited by the clinical resources. Clinical simulators are offering great help to teach the fundamentals of clinical medicine and allow quality teaching when clinical resources are limited.

During the basic sciences, bedside clinical teaching was limited to teach physical diagnosis. The current emphasis is to bring, incrementally, clinical teaching from the very first months of medical school. From the very beginning, a student starts to learn how to obtain a history and how to do the basics of physical findings.

There are some issues to be discussed as we review Caribbean school curriculum and didactic methodology.

- How much detail should be taught in each discipline?

Medical academia is debating this issue, and the divide between clinical sciences faculty and basic science faculty continues. Many would say that some content presented belongs in a PhD curriculum, while others would say that Step 1 should define what students should know and the content should have strong science background needed to learn clinical sciences. And the debate goes on. The National Board of Medical Examiners, which organizes the licensing examinations, could define the depth of content needed by a medical student during the basic science courses. By determining the content of the examination they would make, every school could adjust the teaching accordingly. It is my opinion that the truth may rest in the middle.

The lack of continuum between medical school and residency creates part of the problem. For example, every student needs to know the basic principles of pharmacology, pharmacokinetics, and drug metabolism as well as fundamental types of drugs. If that is taught during the basic sciences, it should be enough to graduate. Teaching and learning should continue during the postgraduate period. If the graduate goes into internal medicine, more knowledge of pharmacology is necessary and should be taught. This should be adjusted for every medical or surgical specialty.

I believe that a continuum of education uniting undergraduate and post-graduate education should exist. Additional teaching should take place during post graduate training. Unfortunately this idea is unrealistic in the way the transition between medical school and postgraduate training takes place, Presently, in medical school, we present so much information that promotes memorization and not reasoning. These people have the rest of their career to learn details, and some details can wait for advanced training!

One of the serious consequences of the current approach—for example, demanding knowledge of hundreds of drugs—is that it leaves not enough time devoted to critical thinking and reasoning. Also, many concepts are taught in an isolated vacuum of a discipline without interaction with other disciplines. The student response to such an approach is raw memorization with little reasoning. That becomes very evident to those who have taught the introductory phases of clinical medicine.

This issue will not be resolved until the NBME explains its expectations clearly and until academic clinicians gain a greater role in the planning of curriculum content. The current trend toward integration of the curriculum is a good first step.

The issue at the moment is to define the best way to teach, promoting what we should teach will be guided by the NBME.

- Does the student population, with a very diverse academic background, learn effectively with a single didactic approach?
- Is the geographic division between a basic science campus with a distributed clinical teaching conducive to the best way to train physicians?
- Are the differences in performance in Step 1 and 2 between students at US schools and Caribbean schools reflection of the teaching, the curriculum, or the students?
- Do licensing examinations serve as an effective tool for comparison between schools? All students take the same examinations regardless of where they were taught. What are the reasons for the consistent differences in results?

Will address these issues separately.

1. Does the student population, with very diverse academic background, learn effectively with a single didactic approach?

Substantial differences existed in the academic background of a Caribbean school class, but everyone was taught the same in the same time. The result was, quite often, that students, especially the weaker ones, memorize to keep up, to use review books and notes without exploring in some depth basic concepts that should serves as the foundation for future learning of clinical medicine. Raw memorization guaranteed that when the time came to put that information to practical clinical application, the information was forgotten or poorly understood.

Fortunately progress is being made as Caribbean schools grow and improve. Recognition that not all students learn the same way or at the same speed is accepted, and formal programs are created to provide support and tutoring to students in need. This was discussed in an earlier chapter.

2. Is the geographic division between a basic science campus and a diversified clinical teaching, as originally designed, conducive to the best way to train physicians?

The traditional organization of Caribbean medical schools had a clear separation between basic science and clinical sciences. The former took place in a Caribbean island and the clinical teaching at a multiplicity of hospitals in the United States and some in England.

The connection between basic science teaching and clinical teaching was very limited. In fact, from a functional perspective, it appeared as if Caribbean schools were two-year medical schools with a distributed clinical program that, at the end of two years granted an MD degree. This organization continues today since, from a regulatory perspective, Caribbean schools are not allowed to teach any basic sciences in the United States.

If one wants to wonder as to why there may be some discrepancies in academic performance between US and Caribbean schools, this geographic separation must be included as one of the factors. It prevents the creation of a cohesive academic atmosphere with participation of both areas in seminars, conferences, or joint projects. But above all, it had shifted the basic science curriculum control to the basic science faculty who decide what are they going to teach and what it is that medical students need to know at a given stage of development. As an example, I have seen a biochemist teaching about Na+ and K+ channels and expanding in detail the clinical conditions that those abnormalities cause. This was taught, to brand-new, fresh, first-year medical students who never heard about arrhythmias or ventricular tachycardia and would not get the basis of electrophysiology until months later!

I have also seen a professor demand one hour of lecture time to cover a very rare disease in the United States, but it was on the professor field of interest. Desire was granted since basic science faculty dominated the curriculum committee and the "club" would not argue with a senior member.

The real discussion should always be what should a physician know that is essential for the quality practice of medicine? Can a group of PhD's alone or in dominance make that decision? The planning of a curriculum requires a balance between clinical and basic science faculty in the composition of a curriculum committee. Unfortunately, the long distances created dominance by basic scientists and now, despite the availability of excellent communication technology, it has not changed the prevalent culture.

- **Are the differences in performance in Step 1 and 2 between students at US schools and Caribbean schools reflection of the teaching, the curriculum, or the students?**

Given the large sample, we can assume that licensing examinations serve as an effective tool for comparison. All students take the same examinations regardless of where they were taught. What are the reasons for the consistent differences in results?

There is no question that there are differences in performance on Step 1 and 2 between US students and Caribbean students. There is no simple answer as to why, and most likely it is a multifactorial problem.

US students show strong similarities in their academic background. But also statistically they are a very tight group. Not only are their college GPAs higher, but more importantly, the standard deviation is quite narrow, giving a more uniform group.

Caribbean students not only have a slightly lower GPA but the standard deviation is much higher, determined by the wide variability in backgrounds, achievements, etc. It is difficult to compare a thirty-five-year-old army medic with years of combat experience who had been out of college for years and now entering medical school to a twenty-three-year-old recent college graduate. There have to be differences.

The answer to this should be simple. If you accept that your students may be different and they have to learn the same material, your teaching methods need to adapt accordingly. This is happening very slowly and needs to continue to happen until results are comparable on Step 1 scores between the two groups, US and Caribbean students. It is the responsibility of the schools to work on the approaches to narrow the differences. This may require changes in class size, different methods, and teaching techniques even if it affects the bottom line. Otherwise Caribbean students will always be handicapped!

How Was Medicine Taught in Caribbean Schools and How Has It Evolved?

From the very beginning, Caribbean medical schools have designed their curriculum to be very similar to that of US medical schools. The basic science component was commonly divided in four semesters, each of approximately fifteen to seventeen weeks. In most schools these semesters are presented with short breaks of two or three weeks. In other words, Caribbean schools were teaching the same material than US schools in shorter semesters, thus in an accelerated, condensed manner. No wonder attrition was high.

This old approach was very beneficial to Caribbean schools since teaching was essentially lecture based, and it made little difference to give a lecture to one hundred students or seven hundred students, provided the classroom had the proper facilities. The content is presented in the same manner for all students without recognizing that not everyone learns the same way. Lecture after lecture for several hours is tiring to the student whose attention span will certainly decrease after several hours.

The lecture approach has been helped with the use of recording technology that allows the student to review the material at his own pace. Stop, repeat, and watch a lecture in total or in part. This technology allows review and repetition, providing the ability to listen to concepts again and again until they are understood (or memorized). This technology is offered in US schools and also in some Caribbean schools.

But part of the problem continued. The transfer of information was one-sided, from the faculty to the students, thinking not required.

The introduction of problem-based learning was one of the first changes that took place in the reform of the didactic approaches.

In a PBL curriculum, the faculty assists students in the research of the case or concepts, the formulation of problems, and the search for supporting data. This method encouraged individual and group thinking, not just unilateral transfer of information like a lecture. The approach of using PBL was applied with varying success in some Caribbean schools.

One of the issues faced by Caribbean schools was the student-faculty ratio. Although PBL-trained facilitators do not have to be experts on the topics, having someone with no knowledge of medicine, disrupts the progress, and can lead students astray in their search of proper and correct information. An uninformed facilitator can mislead students in their independent research and learning.

Caribbean schools have gradually changed, some have maintained the traditional lecture approach, some have kept lot of lectures and added group discussion or PBL methodology. This has led to a trend toward integration of basic science and clinical concepts. Some have had a radical change, moving completely to system integration.

It will take more data gathering and correlation between two approaches to reach valid conclusions and determine that a new system is better than an old system. In some cases change was done without the careful joint work of basic scientists and clinicians together to create true curricular integration. Some have implemented change with almost no clinical involvement with basis scientists, convinced that what they taught was critical and had to protect their turf.

Some US schools have spent years for basic scientists and clinicians to create a truly integrated curriculum and we will have to wait and see if standardized tests show significant changes. On the other hand, we have seen efforts to create an integrated curriculum in a few months resulting in a curriculum that is like the "rearranging the chairs in the Titanic" with the old lectures just being placed in a different order and time. This can result in glaring deficiencies, insufficient time dedicated to dominant diseases, and the lack of any emphasis on prevalent problems in a population.

Another change that deserves mentioning is the increased emphasis on small group discussions, often centered around a case or with the use of a simulator. This is done at the expense of large classroom lecture time. Several Caribbean schools have created outstanding simulator centers that provide a great opportunity to apply many of new methodologies, integration, small groups, and student participation. Teaching around simulators has allowed opportunities for the different teaching approaches to coalesce into one. Again, some of the problems of many Caribbean schools is the low numbers of clinicians who could provide knowledge and experience to a small group discussion and the need for large numbers of small groups to gain the maximum advantage of small-group teaching.

From an educator perspective, the system-based approach is sensible. It allows educators to link together various disciplines and place emphasis on the mechanism of disease and pathophysiology essential for students to have true understanding of a disease and not rely on memorization of symptoms and findings. Once again, time will tell if the application of this method in Caribbean schools leads to performance improvements.

Have these changes resulted in substantial student improvement? The following are some comments extracted from the literature:

- "Students trained within an integrated curriculum made more accurate diagnoses than did students trained in a conventional curriculum."
- "Vertical integration between basic sciences and clinical medicine in problem-based learning curricula stimulated better understanding of biomedical principles than did conventional curricula"

- "A high degree of horizontal integration occurred in the early years, but more input from clinicians was needed throughout the curriculum to achieve vertical integration."

One issue that needs to be raised is the one of creativity. Caribbean schools have, in general, molded the teaching methods around prevailing methods in US schools. There are, however, important differences to recognize and that should go in the planning of a curriculum (some of them we have already discussed):

- A percentage of students come to a Caribbean school with a lower academic background.
- The experienced clinical faculty is relatively small.
- The clinical and basic science are separated by large distances.

This should require that curriculum planning take these factors into consideration and develop methods that are adaptable to the needs and circumstances. For example, the use of video technology should be expanded so more faculty is added. Small groups should be expanded at the expense of large lectures. Regulators may express concern that the use of video-conferencing is distance education instead of considering them supplemental new educational opportunities.

The basic science curriculum, in Caribbean schools needs deep critical review before jumping to conclusions. A critical need is to adopt methods that are special for the Caribbean students. Some will do OK following a US school approach. Others need more time and more tutoring. Schools need to recognize that many of their students may be different, and they need to adjust accordingly. These multifactorial issues make it more difficult to determine which approaches work and which do not.

In a separate section, we will discuss the fifth or extended semester, a period unique to several Caribbean schools. Clinical education will also be discussed in a separate section. Caribbean students, once they pass Step 1, do their clinical training in US hospitals contracted by the school. More about that later.

CHAPTER 14

The COMP

AFTER SUCCESSFUL COMPLETION of all basic sciences courses, how can the schools be sure that students can pass the Step 1 of the US licensing examinations? How can students know what their strengths and weaknesses are? Do they need special preparation and review?

The National Board of Medical Examiners considered these issues and prepared an examination that allows students and schools to evaluate the preparedness of their students.

NBME offers a Comprehensive Basic Science Examination that allows students to evaluate their readiness to take the demanding Step 1 test. Starting in 2001 some Caribbean schools dictated that students had to take and pass this comprehensive examination before they proceed to Step 1.

The NBME Comprehensive examination is offered by the board as a review examination. The COMP is used by more than thirty US schools and a number of Caribbean schools. As per the NBME "It consists of 184 multiple-choice questions and associated pictures. It is administered during a four (4) hour and fifteen (15) minute session. The examination is divided into four 60-minute sessions."

The passing score of the COMP can change based on Step 1 passing score and is adjusted to maintain a useful correlation with Step 1.

The Comprehensive Basic Science Examination content outline includes questions on the following areas:

- General Principles 25%
- Individual Organ Systems 75%
    - Hematopoietic and Lymphoreticular

- Central and Peripheral Nervous System
- Skin and relate connective tissue
- Musculoskeletal
- Respiratory
- Cardiovascular
- Gastrointestinal
- Renal/Urinary
- Reproductive
- Endocrine
- Immune

- Process
  - Normal 25–45%
  - Abnormal 30–50%
  - Principles of Therapeutics.................................. 15–35%
- Psychosocial, cultural and environmental considerations....10%

(Source: National Board of Medical Examiners)

The COMP consists mainly of questions retired from previous Step 1 examinations, and it offers students a very valuable tool to establish their readiness to pass Step 1. The COMP and Step 1 scores have maintained a very good statistical correlation, allowing a reasonable prediction of how well a student will do when taking Step 1, That is one of the reasons why some schools require passing the COMP with a predetermined score before they allow the students to sit for Step 1. Simultaneously many schools have established the policy that COMP scores will not be part of the official transcript thus concealing how many times students had to take the examination.

Passing the COMP on the first trial is usually limited to approximately 50% of students or less. About 98% pass it after three trials. As expected, those with better performance during basic sciences courses have a higher likelihood of passing the COMP the first time. Those who have to take it up to three times clearly indicate lacking adequate knowledge and will require much longer review and preparation before taking Step 1. Some school dismiss a student after three or four failures, and others let them take as many times as they want, but they will have to do their preparation on their own.

Some critics and accrediting agencies have indicated that existing school policies regarding passing the COMP before being allowed to take Step 1 is one way for schools to distort true Step 1 statistics. If students have to take the COMP two or three times, it impacts the credibility of statements such as, "Our first-time passing rate for Step 1 is 90% or 95%." While mathematically correct, it does not report on attempts to pass the COMP before being allowed to sit for Step 1. Some think that if you have to take the COMP three times, it is equivalent to have taken Step 1 more than once, but this information is not shared.

Since the COMP is taken shortly after completion of basic science courses, failure to pass the COMP on a first trial often indicates that the time frame between the end of basic sciences was too short for an adequate review of earlier material. Failing the COMP three times indicates serious lack of knowledge and preparation. Presenting both numbers—first-time passing and attempts of the COMP—gives a more realistic presentation of the academic performance of students in a specific school. It will have an impact on residency placement since program directors will add this data to further identify weak students. Marketing, however, would not like that since they place a high value on Step 1 passing percentages without mentioning the COMP. This obviously can help the very weak students.

Issues raised around the COMP deserve several comments.

- First, in the eyes of some accreditors, the COMP is a tool to create a false high percentage of students passing Step 1 since it excludes those who have completed the necessary courses to take Step 1 but are held back by their COMP scores.
- The COMP gives the student a realistic view of the level of preparation and tells them when they are likely to pass Step 1.
- By giving students multiple opportunities to take the COMP before the student is eligible for academic dismissal, it distorts the true statistics of attrition.

- When schools report a certain percentage passing Step 1 on the first trial, they do not report how many times a student took the COMP.
- There are other tests similar to the NBME COMP offered by private vendors, but essentially they are used for the same purpose as the COMP.

In summary, use of the COMP has provided a good assessment before students move to directly to Step 1. Students often complain that they do not have enough time to prepare, but the fact is that it provides students with information regarding their areas of strength and weaknesses.

CHAPTER 15

Caribbean Schools and a Fifth Semester

APPROXIMATELY FIFTEEN YEARS ago, Caribbean schools started incorporating a fifth semester as a transitional phase between the end of basic education and the start of clinical education. Directors of medical education and program directors reported that a distinct difference in the clinical skills between students in Caribbean schools and their counterparts coming from US medical schools.

What are the reasons for differences? Many reasons were postulated and we will mention some:

- The very limited exposure to clinical situations and their lack of knowledge of American hospital operations and routines
- Difference in the teaching of Introduction to Clinical Medicine and the teaching of mechanisms of disease
- Teaching of physical examination techniques inadequate
- Students self-confidence when abruptly encountering clinical situations in a technologically overwhelming US hospital

The true reasons were not known, but it was probably a multifactorial problem. This created a disadvantage for the Caribbean students when exposed constantly to their US counterparts. The level of deficiencies were broad ranging, from quality of physical examination to medical record-keeping accompanied by some lack of self-confidence.

Because of these reported differences and in an effort to improve Caribbean student performance in clinical situations and in NBME examinations as well as their chances of securing residency, a decision was made by several schools to start a transitional program between the basic sciences component and the start of the clinical training and clerkships. This represented a fifth semester, and in most cases, it was conducted in the United States although some schools maintained such programs in the country where basic sciences were taught.

Schools organized the curriculum for this fifth semester in different ways, but from a regulatory perspective, they could not offer any basic science teaching and had to concentrate on clinical sciences. Fortunately one could review concepts on the pathophysiology of a disease and the relationship with basic science concepts within the discussion of a clinical case. The sessions offered some basic and clinical science integration and gave the opportunity to review some important basic science concepts related to the disease process under discussion as seen from a clinician perspective.

Each school that created a fifth semester developed a different curriculum based on their views of what was best for the students. The following are some common aspects of the curriculum of the fifth semesters as it developed in the various schools.

- Lecture series covering a diversity of clinical topics. These lectures covered, in more advanced clinical depth, some topics that what were already presented in the basic science courses or added new topics that could not be discussed previous semesters because of lack of time. The lectures were usually discussed by a specialist and were almost always case based, presented at a level closer to that of lectures to residents.
- In addition, lectures were presented on special topics not well covered in the island. For example initial aspects of geriatrics, medical aspects of substance abuse, review of statistics, legal aspects of medical practice, etc.
- Small-group sessions that presented a clinical case and were structured as an interactive session with questions and answers and active student participation, mimicking teaching rounds.
- For those schools that had established simulator centers, cases were presented, and the students had to work the case on the

simulator and observe the physiological changes. These sessions were tutored by clinicians or teaching assistants and provided for very lively discussions on how to handle different medical emergencies and many other issues of practical application during hospital clerkships.

- The fifth semester provided an opportunity to review and practice pf physical examination techniques that represent an important component of Step 2-CS (clinical skills).
- The fifth semester also provided the opportunity to focus on patient interview and doctor-patient communication. Standardized patients were often used for this type of activity.
- Medical record preparation, including history and physicals and SOAP notes.
- Clinical sessions in physician offices or emergency departments. At this point students had minimal clinical experience, so they were given opportunities to interview, examine, and discuss actual clinical cases.
- Other sessions and topics that varied from program to program.

Students often expressed negative thoughts and often stated that this semester existed only to collect additional tuition and delay their graduation. Some of this became part of the folklore that appeared in student blogs or websites., Having taught in this semester, I observed that it narrowed the gap between US and Caribbean students. After they completed the semester, students were able to appreciate how much better prepared they were to enter a busy clinical clerkship.

In summary, this fifth semester—which lasted from six weeks to twelve weeks, according to schools—allowed students to transfer with greater confidence into the clinical environment.

In my opinion, the fifth semester gave students not only an improved foundation of knowledge but also gave them greater confidence when placed in a clinical setting working side by side with students from other schools. The increased use of simulators has created new opportunities to teach the initial aspects of clinical medicine in a well-controlled environment. Cases created for use with a simulator allow realistic situations and permits the evaluation of student's critical thinking and decision making.

CHAPTER 16

USMLE Step 1

THE NATIONAL BOARD of Medical Examiners (NBME), administers in the United States all three phases of the licensing process and the examination is recognized by all fifty states. The NBME was created in 1915 as an independent, nonprofit organization whose stated mission is to "protect the health of the public through state of the art assessment of health professionals."

Prior to the World War II and until the early sixties, states administered their own exams, and gave reciprocity to physicians who had passed other state exams. Subsequently, states began to use the results of an NBME exam and that permitted students to take only one examination in order to obtain a license.

The United States Medical Licensing Examination, or USMLE, is offered by the National Board of Medical Examiners and the Federation of State Medical Boards (FSMB) and was introduced in 1992. These examinations are mandatory in order for a physician to be licensed to practice medicine in a state.

In the life of medical students Step 1 of the United States Licensing Examination is the first real hurdle in the quest to become a licensed physician in the US. Step 1 is the first of three examinations taken at the end of the basic science courses. Step 2 is taken during the clinical clerkships and consist of two parts, clinical knowledge and clinical skills. Step 3 is taken during the first year of residency. Everyone, US students and international graduates alike, who seeks to obtain a license to practice medicine in the US must undergo this arduous process.

USMLE examinations should be the great equalizer in the testing of knowledge for everyone, and its results are important pieces of data used by program directors in the ranking of applicants for residence. Its scores are of practical use in comparing education at all medical schools worldwide and are commonly used to evaluate Caribbean schools in comparison to US schools.

The USMLE describes Step 1 as follows:

> An eight-hour computer-based test taken in a single-day, composed of seven 44-question sections with a total of 308 multiple-choice questions· One hour is provided for each section, allotting an average of a minute and eighteen seconds to answer each question.
>
> Step 1 is designed to test the knowledge learned during the basic science years of medical school. This includes anatomy, behavioral sciences, biochemistry, microbiology, pathology, pharmacology, and physiology. In addition to the above, the examination includes interdisciplinary areas such as genetics, aging, immunology, nutrition, and molecular and cell biology as well as epidemiology, and medical ethics. Each exam is dynamically generated for each test taker; while the general proportion of questions derived from a particular subject is the same, some test takers report that certain subjects are either emphasized or deemphasized.
>
> Examinees receive results as a three-digit score and a two-digit score; the latter of which is not a percentile. The three-digit score is a scaled score with a mean that fluctuates test year to test year, and a standard deviation of approximately 21.The three-digit score is calculated using a statistical percentile that ensures that scores from different years are read on a common scale, since the exam is known to get progressively more difficult as the years go on. However, the NBME does not disclose how this three-digit score is calculated. The two digit score is a scaled score that defines 75 as the minimum passing score, which is equivalent to a 192 on the three-digit scale.

The three-digit score is more commonly used. In 2014, the national mean score was 229 with a standard deviation of 20; the minimum passing score was 192. Many residency programs use a cutoff score for Step 1, usually between 210 and 220, below which applicants are unlikely to be considered. Many residency programs will not interview a student who has failed Step 1 and had to retake the examination. These are critical concepts, and it needs to be drilled into medical students that passing is not enough, the score will play a significant role in determining the future. In student lingo, they "need to nail it."

Scores distribution, as presented by the National Board of Medical Examiners, is shown below. In 2014, 15,149 US MD graduates took the examination for the first time, and 812 were repeaters. Also, 2,746 DOs sat for this examination together with 18,038 international medical graduates (including graduates of Caribbean schools), and of these, 2,889 were repeaters. The results are of interest and are shown in the following table.

Table 14-1

	% Passing
US or Canadian students	
1st time takers	96%
Repeaters	68%
Doctors of Osteopathy	
1st time takers	93%
Repeaters	69%
International Graduates	
1st time takers	78%
Repeaters	39%

Source: National Board of Medical Examiners 2014

Some Caribbean schools report that 90% or more of their students pass Step 1 on a first attempt. They do not indicate, however, that the data they report represent, one year result or an average of three years Failure to define the denominator that allows calculation of the percentage obfuscates the interpretation of the data. In the absence of an independent report, this data cannot be questioned, but it would be useful to have an independent source to confirm the data coming from individual schools.

In the absence of any supporting audited information provided by an independent organization, we have decided not to provide individual school information unless it is externally validated. This may be unfair to some schools that provide accurate data, but we decided to apply the same principle to all.

We will try to identify the potential reasons why international medical graduates underperform US graduates in these licensing examinations. The reasons and factors could be many.

- For Caribbean graduates, the basic science information is presented in a compact manner and memorization is common practice. Doing a large part of your learning from class handouts and practice questions can decrease deductive reasoning. For many students, sixteen weeks to learn, for example, physiology or pharmacology is not enough, unless you just memorize answers without concept understanding. That is obvious when you ask students to reason and calculate something as simple as pulmonary resistance or the application of the Fick principle. Some will do it very well. Many cannot remember the principle to apply.
- Another potential reason is that during the course, the facultycreate questions for periodic testing that do not follow a format used by the USMLE and students do not have real practice on STEP 1 format of questions. Some schools are trying to do exam questions in a precise USMLE format so students get some practice with questions similar to the ones they will encounter in Step 1. When this happens in all schools, results are likely to improve.
- English as a second language is another issue for many. Reading large stems, the introductory part of the question, consumes

time and may slow you down if English understanding is limited.

- Many international graduates were never exposed to multiple-choice questions. It requires practice.
- Finally, a group of international students take the examination years after graduating from medical school, and in many cases, it is like starting medical school all over again.

How long students study in preparation for the examination? It is a demanding examination that will play a significant role in the student's career. The time spent preparing for this examination is substantial. Seventy three (73) percent will spend between six and twelve months, and only 26% will feel confident with less than three months of preparation.

For Caribbean schools, there are several alternatives to improve Step 1 statistics and they will be discussed separately.

Some schools place their emphasis in preparing students to pass Step 1 at the expense of a well-grounded scientific education. If you mainly teach to answer questions, you do not have any guarantees that students truly learned the material. How much of the correct answering of Step 1 comes from raw memorization through the use of question books? Does that mean that the student knows the material? Or are they trained to remember concepts often not tied together in a logical manner.

Is Step 1 a good parameter to compare schools? A difficult question to answer. We know the numbers, and we know that US students score higher on average than Caribbean students. All I am willing to say that they score better on an examination. It will take a lot more to determine who is better prepared in the knowledge of medicine.

CHAPTER 17

USMLE Step 2

STEP 2 OF the USMLE is taken during the clinical training period, usually in the senior year, and is divided into two components: clinical knowledge (CK) and clinical skills (CS). All Caribbean students, must take Step 2 CS and Step 2 CK prior to applying for residency in the United States, and they cannot begin residency without successfully completing both components.

Step 2 evaluates the application of medical knowledge, skills, and the understanding of clinical science essential for the provision of patient care under supervision.

Step 2-CK is a nine-hour-long, single-day computer-based examination that assesses through, multiple-choice questions medical knowledge and understanding of clinical science. It consists of 340–355 questions divided into eight sets. Students are allowed no more than forty-five minutes per set of forty-five questions.

The test is administered at **Prometric** testing sites. The company also administers Medical the College Admission Test (MCAT) and operates testing sites in 160 countries.

Step 2 (CK) scoring is reported in three-digit scores. The mean score for first-time examinees is in the range of 220–230, and the recommended minimum passing score is 209. Overall, US senior applicants had mean USMLE Step 2 scores of 242.0 (s.d. = 16.6) and independent applicants (including Caribbean students) had mean scores of 227.0 (s.d. = 18.9).

Step 2 Clinical Skills (CS) is administered to medical students or graduates who wish to become licensed physicians in the United States. Students take the examination during their fourth year of medical school. The examination consists of standardized patient encounters in which the student takes a history, does a physical examination, determines differential diagnoses, and then writes a patient note The topics covered are common outpatient or emergency room visits that are encountered in the fields of internal medicine, surgery, psychiatry, pediatrics, and obstetrics and gynecology. Examinees are expected to investigate the simulated patient's chief complaint, as well as obtain a thorough assessment of their past medical history, medications, allergies, social history (including alcohol, tobacco, drug use, sexual practices, etc.), and family history.

The examination consists of three parts.

- **Integrated Clinical Encounter (ICE)** evaluates the ability to collect pertinent clinical information from the SP and to write an appropriate patient note with differential after the clinical encounter.
- **Communication and Interpersonal Skills (CIS)** evaluates the question-asking skills (asking open-ended questions, information-sharing skills, and professionalism.
- **Spoken English Proficiency (SEP)** evaluates clarity of spoken English communication, pronunciation, word choice, and minimizing the need to repeat questions or statements.

Examinees are allowed fifteen minutes to complete each encounter and ten minutes to write the patient note. The examinees will report up to three related differential diagnoses relating and determine tests or procedures needed. Over the course of an eight-hour exam day, the examinees complete twelve such encounters.

The test is graded on a pass-fail basis, in order to pass the examination, one must achieve a grade of "Pass" in each of the three subcomponents.

The enclosed table show Step 2 CK results for different cohorts of students.

Table 15-1. Summary of Step 2 CK Results

	% Passing
US or Canadian students	
1st-Time Takers	97%
Repeaters	70%
Doctors of Osteopathy	
1st-Time Takers	95%
Repeaters	68%
International Graduates	
1st-Time Takers	80%
Repeaters	39%

The following is a table depicting average Step 2 scores for students graduated from US schools and the cohort of international graduates (including Caribbean graduates) matching and not matching in different specialties.

Table 15-2

	Matched		**Not Matched**	
Step 2 Scores	**US Grads**	**US IMG**	**US Grads**	**US IMG**
Anesthesiology	241	238	223	212
Emer. Medicine	243	235	225	223
Family Medicine	234	213	216	203
Internal Med.	243	228	219	210
Neurology	241	222	236	206
Ob-Gyn	242	232	225	213
Pathology	241	226	236	206
Pediatrics	241	224	219	208
Phys. Med. & Rehab	234	231	220	212
Psychiatry	233	211	216	202

Radiology	249	241	236	223
Surgery-General	245	234	226	216

Source: www.doctorsintraining.com/blog/usmle2-ck-averag

As was the case for the Step 1 scores, the students who obtain a residency in more competitive specialties have higher average Step 2 scores. International medical graduates, even those who match in more competitive specialties, score lower than US graduates.

The NRMP released updated results on the 2014 Main Residency Match. Step 2 CK score averages were highest in those that matched in dermatology, otolaryngology, plastic surgery, orthopedic surgery and vascular surgery, and they all were in the 250s.

The following is obtained from information given by the USMLE concerning passing percentage of test takers, for each of the three subcomponents mentioned above.

Table 15-3

		2013–2014	
	ICE	**CIS**	**SEP**
All US/Canadian Schools	97%	98%	>99%
All Non-US/ Canadian Schools	81%	89%	97%

Source: USMLE

As stated earlier, Step 1 and Step 2 demonstrate that US students score better than their counterparts. The factors causing that are multiple and have already been discussed. Since these results are the only objective data in the hands of program directors, it is clear as to why they would show preference for US graduates. It is the responsibility of Caribbean schools to create teaching methods that will equalize the results. If this happens, the Caribbean graduate would have improved performance in the NRMP match.

CHAPTER 18

Clinical Training

UNTIL RECENTLY, THE first two years of medical school, done in a Caribbean island, consisted primarily of basic science lectures and all clinical teaching was done in the United States. Very little clinical medicine was taught in the initial two years with the exception of physical diagnosis and a semester of introduction to clinical medicine with very little practical teaching.

It has been like that since the start of Caribbean education, in part because that it was the way US medical school did things and in part resulting from regulatory decisions by the Department of Education not to allow basic science teaching in the United States. From a practical perspective, the lack of regular interaction between basic and clinical faculty was as if you were operating two different schools controlled by a central administrative office whose staff neither taught basic or clinical sciences.

Times have changed, and gradually, basic and clinical sciences are offered with an integrated approach, in some schools starting from the first semester. The trends are similar to the current trends in US schools, once again demonstrating that Caribbean schools did not design curricula to meet the needs of the students but just replicated what was happening in US schools.

Caribbean schools needed to do clinical teaching in the United States (with the exceptions of few clerkships in the UK) for multiple reasons.

- Most students planned to practice in the United States, so they needed to be exposed to clinical teaching in the United States as well as the US health-care system.

- Most islands do not have sufficient clinical resources to accommodate the large class size common in the Caribbean model.
- The Caribbean hospital systems (with rare exceptions) are not modern enough to provide an education comparable to what is offered in a US hospital.

The number of students moving from the Caribbean to the United States for clinical training necessitated the creation of a distributed model of education involving multiple hospitals. US schools did not have experience with this model since most schools used, at best, a handful of hospitals to train their students. The only exception I know that truly operates a distributed model of clinical education is the Uniformed Services University of the Health Sciences that uses multiple military hospitals.

The diversified clinical training created, for Caribbean schools, its own set of issues.

- It was very difficult to create any standardization on curriculum and teaching. The people doing the clinical teaching were in different hospitals, different systems, or different cities.
- Most of the time, the clinical teachers did not have a faculty appointments in the school.
- There was little oversight of the quality of teaching since it was difficult to evaluate each site and each clerkship on a regular and timely basis.
- Hospitals often contracted with other offshore schools or had students from US medical schools. That made it very difficult to create a curriculum for one school that could be applied to all hospitals where students rotated.
- Students rotated in multiple hospitals and in multiple cities. This often created inconveniences for the students who had to move from place to place every few weeks since many hospitals offered only one clerkship. In addition to the complexity of moving from place to place, it precluded them from establishing

long-term relationships with physicians who could serve as mentors and be of help in securing residencies.

- The number of available clinical sites often made it difficult to create a seamless schedule for each student. Students may have to wait even up to several weeks until openings were available for certain clerkships. This eroded the concept of an accelerated program.
- Evaluation of students was decentralized, each hospital and teaching physician submitting grades and evaluations independently, often very late. It made the identification of students with academic issues a very difficult task.
- A regulatory and accreditation requirement was that all clinical rotations be conducted in a hospital with ACGME-approved residencies. Some regulatory loophole allowed that clerkships be offered where there was no residency in a specific field. For example, a family practice residency provided the justification to offer an OB or surgical clerkship in those hospitals. Simply said, it is a complex system with multiple ways to comply or not to comply with the regulations regarding accreditation or for state medical licensing.
- LCME regulations do not allow for Caribbean students to do clerkships or electives in universities' programs. This limited the potential of developing clerkship sites. For example, a well-recognized nonuniversity teaching hospital linked to a medical school that for years had matched a school's graduates would not take students for clerkships because of its feared LCME regulations. These rules appear very protective, punishing students from the potential of getting a good clinical rotation.

Some general observations can be made about the hospitals where Caribbean students do their clinical training.

- Some hospitals are well-known teaching hospitals with long-standing tradition and quality of education.

- The majority of the institutions are community hospitals with little, if any, dedicated full-time faculty, with most of the teaching done by practicing physicians on a voluntary basis.
- Some hospitals have created a revenue source by taking students from several Caribbean schools. At $300–$500 dollars per students per week, it creates a good source of funds to supplement a budget. As a consequence, often too many students from several schools are rotating at the same time—too many for the clinical material available—and students get a mediocre education. It is for that reason that some schools canceled contracts with these institutions.
- Students from US schools may rotate through the same hospital. This has certain advantages, exposing Caribbean students to students from other schools. This helps Caribbean students since they see that they perform as well as their US counterparts. This is a common comment by Caribbean students.
- The size and quality of the house staff in the various residencies may vary. Since, from a practical perspective, residents do a substantial amount of the bedside teaching, this may affect the quality of education. Good residents imply good bedside teaching.

Lack of standardized data makes it impossible to evaluate the quality of teaching and education in the multiple hospitals used by the distributed model used by Caribbean schools. To our knowledge, currently, there are no criteria or accepted accreditation standards to guarantee a similar quality education at all clinical training sites. Each accrediting agency approves the school without specified criteria evaluating the clinical site where the students are trained.

Some pertinent questions that accrediting agencies could ask of each training site during an accreditation visit could include the following:

- Are sufficient clerkships readily available, or might the student have hiatuses in their education because not enough rotations are available and they have to wait weeks or months for the next rotation?

- In each hospital where students rotate, what is the ratio of residents to students, and how many students are in a ward team?
- How many ACGME-approved residencies are in each hospital? Hospitals with a single ACGME residency and several clerkships should not be approved.
- What is the ratio of US graduates versus international medical graduates? This may sound unfair and elitist; however, it is realistic. If a teaching hospital attracts US graduates, it is a well-known reflection of the reputation of the institution.
- Are the director of medical education, department chairs, and faculty full-time or part-time? This could indicate the hospitals' support of medical education and the support available to students.
- Are the physician-teachers full-time or part-time, and what is the ratio between full-time and part-time? This could also be interpreted as an elitist perception; however, it could indicate the amount of time that a physician could devote to students.
- What is the board passing percentage of residents in various affiliated hospital? This is an indirect evaluator of the quality of teaching at a given hospital.
- How many students are in each clerkship in a given month and how many students are in a house staff team? This is important with hospitals that have contracted with several schools. Too many students in a house staff team will dilute the educational experience.

A criticism of Caribbean medical schools is that the clinical preparation of its students is not at par with their US counterparts. The only objective parameter available is performance on licensing examinations that reflect their clinical knowledge and skills. The table below shows Step 1 and 2 scores for NRMP matched students.

Table 16-1

	US US tudents	US IMGs	Non-US IMG
Step 1	230	217	233
Step 2	243	224	227

The same data is shown for those three groups of students that failed to match in 2014.

Table 16-2

	US Students	US IMGs	Non-US IMG
Step 1	221	204	213
Step 2	231	209	218

Source "Charting Outcomes in the Match Characteristics of Applicants Who Matched to Their Preferred Specialty in the 2014 Residency" and "Charting Outcomes in the Match International Medical Graduates Characteristics of Applicants Who Matched to Their Preferred Specialty in the 2013 Main Residency Match" prepared by the American Associations of Medical Colleges

Unfortunately, similar data is not public for Step 2 CS, which tests clinical skills. As shown earlier, Step 2 CK, which tests knowledge and clinical reasoning, shows a difference between US and US IMG students. We could postulate that the reason for the differences, are a carryover from Step 1, which tested basic science. We could also postulate that it may be a reflection of clinical training. It is difficult to reach conclusions until Step 2 data for different training sites is made available. Analysis is also a complex study since one would have to assure that student allocation is random and that better students are not allocated to special sites.

The timely availability of training sites is in some cases a real issue. It has not been uncommon for students to have to wait for weeks for availability of a slot to do one of the required clerkships. For students, that is disappointing and frustrating since it delays graduation and slows their rhythm and may require explanation when applying to residencies. This is a reflection of planning by school administration. It says to me that class size planning does not take into account the availability of clinical resources. For this reason, we suggested above that this information be public and part of the accreditation of the school and the approval of an institution as a training site.

Over the last few years, changes have happened in clinical training offered by Caribbean schools. Some schools have worked in creating several clinical sites in the same geographic area or creating several clerkships in one hospital. This is a major improvement. From the student perspective, it means that they can establish themselves in one region of the country for the duration of their clinical training. From a teaching perspective, it allows the creation of different educational opportunities and establishes the image of a clinical campus. This will go a long way not only to improve education but to improve the reputation of the institution.

Schools have made sustained efforts to increase the number of clinical training sites. This has created competition between Caribbean schools and, potentially, also competition with US schools. The growth of US medical schools' class sizes, as well as the number of new schools and osteopathic schools, have started to create problems and keen competition for teaching sites.

Caribbean schools have for many years compensated hospitals on a per-student basis per week. Currently it is up to $500 per week. This has become very attractive to the often financially stretched hospital, especially those urban and inner city hospitals. US medical schools have used those hospitals for the same purpose and now run the risk of being displaced by Caribbean students. A good example of the developing competition is, as reported by the *New York Times* in December 2010, the request by New York Medical Schools, to protect their access to these teaching sites in view of a contract between Saint George's University School of Medicine and New York hospitals for $100 million, to secure clerkship rotations in their hospitals.

This issue is not new. For many years Caribbean schools have paid hospitals to allow their students do clinicl rotations at their hospitals. As the number of Caribbean schools increases, the need of more sites grew. The payment to the hospitals continued to increase. It is not difficult to do the calculation and understand the reason why some hospitals have contracted with more than one school, sometimes, overcrowding the rotations to the point that some schools terminated the agreement. The development of accrediting criteria applicable to hospitals, as mentioned earlier, will resolve this issue.

The above example is likely to repeat itself elsewhere and the competition will continue. US schools will have to develop different initiatives to retain these hospitals, or they are going to face either a shortage of places or an increased cost that will be associated with an increase in tuition. This is already mentioned by the AAMC in a report on issues regarding clinical training sites. In a recent survey (2015) answered by 83% of US medical schools, the report stated that schools felt "increasing pressure about the availability of clerkship/clinical training sites, particularly new training sites." The same report stated "more than 70% of respondents indicated that developing new sites is more difficult than two years ago." Of interest is to note that only 11% of the schools responding pay money per student to one or more community based sites. This is contrary to Caribbean schools that traditionally have paid the sites or the 71% of DO schools that report paying. LCME accredited schools will have to evaluate alternatives.

The issue is to become more complicated in multiple parts of the United States. The following are the potential factors:

- Medicare, a substantial provider of funds for graduate medical education, has provided only small increments in the number of positions funded. Indirectly this affects how many medical students can be trained in a facility.
- Training, especially in family practice and internal medicine, has evolved toward more ambulatory care training. At present training in an ambulatory setting receives no Medicare funding. For this reason, supporting ambulatory clinical sites for education is complicated. This is a very real and current issue that organized medicine is trying to resolve with the Center for Medicare and Medicaid and with the US Congress.

- Many hospitals, especially urban ones, are not in a financial position to provide adequate support for medical education.
- Existing US medical schools, at the request of AAMC, have increased class size and are in need of more training positions. Some claim they cannot increase enrollment further because of the limitation imposed by the available number of clinical sites.
- The demand for clinical sites will continue to rise as new MD schools as well as DO schools appear and existing ones increase class size. In that environment, Caribbean schools that continue to grow to meet their financial goals will meet a very competitive environment.
- In this scenario, the almighty dollar appears and the scene is set. Supply of training sites is not easy to expand. Demand continues to increase. Existing funding limited. Experience taught that many hospitals have negotiated lucrative contracts with offshore schools. Why not do the same with US schools? US school say that they cannot afford it and would have to increase tuition. Negotiations could begin. After all, students training in a hospital use resources and, hence, cost money. US medical schools should approach this as a business, and supply and demand will determine how much hospitals should be paid. Why differentiate between US and Caribbean schools?

CHAPTER 19

Postgraduate Training—the Match

GRADUATION FROM MEDICAL school is only one step in the career development of new physicians. Postgraduate education is the next critical step. Everyone must do at least an internship to get a license to practice medicine and most graduates do a residency. On "match day" new graduates will determine if they have obtained a position as a resident in a teaching hospital. The process creates its own March madness, every medical student is anxiously waiting for the day in middle of March when they are going to receive a communication as to the outcome of this painful process. "Did I match?" and "Where did you match?" are the only conversations you will hear in schools and hospitals around March 15t Student life is, at that time, in the hands of the computers of the National Residency Matching Program.

The NRMP was created in 1952, Prior to that date, the process was informal, and hospitals attempted to recruit their quota of interns as soon as possible, creating a complicated and often unfair system. The NRMP process has been subject of litigation but survived, unchanged, several attempts. Its software is complicated but fair and is usually in favor of the student. Until then, the process was operated in a decentralized, competitive market. Hospitals benefited from filling their positions as early as possible, and applicants benefited from delaying acceptance of positions. All of it creating a process. unorganized and confusing.

Most US graduates participate on the match. To participate, those graduating from a Caribbean schools, like all other international graduates must have a certificate from the Educational Council of Foreign Medical Graduates (ECFMG certification). In order to obtain the certificate the student must have passed USMLE Step 1, USMLE Step 2 Clinical Knowledge and USMLE Step 2 Clinical Skills and provide a diploma. Most Caribbean schools take care of these details in order for students to be able to participate in the match in a timely manner.

The results of the match are critical for a new graduate career. Failing to match through the NRMP means that the graduate has to seek unfilled positions. The NRMP has now streamlined the process for those who failed to match and who need to find unfilled positions. For students who did not obtain a position on match day, the next step is to enter the NRMP's Supplemental Offer and Acceptance Program (SOAP). Previously, and appropriately, referred to as the "scramble," SOAP offers unmatched students a last chance to match into any unfilled residency positions for that year.

The other option available for recent graduates is to accept a position "outside the match," even before match day. Although this option will guarantee the graduate a residency, it is usually in a noncompetitive institution. Residency programs that did not fill their quota on the match on previous year accept to hire interns before match day. Accepting a position "outside the match" may appear very glamorous for some and exciting for the student. Depending on the student's career desire, it may have some negative consequences. These hospitals that take students "outside the match" are not at the top of the academic hierarchy, and if the student decides to pursue a subspecialty fellowship after residency, chances getting a competitive fellowship will decrease,

IMGs and FMGs make up the majority of SOAP applicants, but USMGs are still favored in this process as well. In 2014, USMGs matched into 609 of the 998 (61%) available positions, leaving only 309 (31%) PGY-1 positions for the 6000+ unmatched IMGs and FMGs. The chances of an IMG graduate to secure a residency through this process is 1 in 20.

One conclusion can be reached. If a student has a very weak medical school record, low Step 1 score, or has failed Step 1 or 2 once and is offered a position" outside the match," take it. The chances of matching are very low and is better to have a residency than having to wait another year, when possibilities are even lower.

How well Caribbean school graduates do in the match? Multiple factors affect the outcome.

- Step 1 and Step 2 scores.
- Important also is the attitude of the institution in regard to foreign graduates. Some institutions have a distinct dislike for them and refuse even to consider them.
- Another major factor is how competitive the medical or surgical specialty is. US graduates will most likely be ranked above international graduates.
- How well does the graduate do interviews? Practice interviews offered by someone with experience has helped the student.
- How well-advised was the student in preparing for the interview process, and how competitive is the candidate for the hospitals he wants to apply to? The student should be advised that the list of hospitals he submits must be compatible with his qualifications.
- The desire by some to enter a couples match or confine themselves to a specific city.

The match is not a precise scientific process. The people ranking the students act on their opinions and biases, sometimes bypassing a good candidate because they may have had, in previous years, bad experiences with graduates of that school, or they may rank high a below-average graduate because he comes from a favorite school. Although the match program is designed to bend in the direction of the student the ranking preferences is decided by the residency program. Programs look at how far down the match list they go, meaning how many students they had to rank in order to fill all of their spots. This is a simple assessment of their recruiting abilities. The best outcome, almost impossible, would be for a program to rank 10 students, and all of them match to their hospital. The other extreme would be a program that ranks 200 applicants and ends with many unfilled positions.

It is easier to understand the complexity of the match and the chances of Caribbean graduates by evaluating the data available, as given by the National Residency Matching Program. Let's start by showing how many positions are available for new graduates, also known as first-year postgraduates or PG-1.

The number of PG-1 positions available through the NRMP are shown in the enclosed table and the following should be noted.

Table 17-1

Year	2011	2012	2013	2014	2015
# Positions	23,410	24,005	26,135	26,678	27,293
Change		595	2,130	543	615
%change		2.47	8.7	2.07	2.03

Source: National Residency Matching Program 2015

In the last five years,

- the number of PG1 positions has increased by about 16%,
- the number of US graduates applying for residency has increased by 9.1%,
- the total number of applicants (including all IMGs) has increased by 9.86%, and
- **the number of US citizens who are international graduates (mainly Caribbean schools graduates) increased by 21.18%.**

These changes would suggest that for Caribbean graduates, the increase in the number of graduates is likely to make the match more competitive.

The sources of graduates is as follows:

Number of Applicants for PG1 Positions

Table 17-2

	2011	2012	2013	2014	2015
US Graduates	16,893	16,875	17,758	17,767	18,447
Previous Graduates	1,766	1,761	1,768	1,861	1,830
DO Graduates	3,142	3,450	3,627	3,768	4,021
Canadian Med School	28	38	34	24	38
Graduates 5th Pathway	20	30	35	50	80
Non US International graduates	10,118	10,004	10,004	9,882	10060
US citizens, international graduates	5708	6249	6882	6952	6917
Total Applicants	37675	38407	40108	40304	41393

Source. National Residency Matching Program 2015

NRMP has published some match data for 2013, including some Caribbean schools (did not find newer data). This is shown below.

Table 17-3

	Ross U.	St. Georges	AUA	SABA	AUC	UMHS
Matched	532	534	180	45	189	85
Unmatched	248	258	207	33	120	103
Total	780	792	387	78	309	188
% Matched	**68.2**	**67.4**	**46.5**	**57.7**	**61.2**	**45.2**

This data, albeit incomplete, is the data published by AAMC and NRMP. Schools often publish their own data, and their numbers often disagree with this data. They may report match rates sometimes as high as mid 80%, and this may be correct for very few Caribbean schools. One common problem with school-provided data is the failure to define the denominator. For example, schools that claim matching 80%, is that 80% a one-time event? Is that the average for two, three years? How can you trust a percentage if you do not know the denominator? Also, schools will describe as "matched" those that secured a residency without going through the match, and the NRMP official data will include only those who match through the NRMP. These are reasons why I do not use school-specific data in our presentation.

From NRMP data we can conclude the following:

- 96% of US graduates secure a residency through the match.
- Graduates from Caribbean schools' match rate ranges from 68% to 47%. (although some schools report higher numbers).
- Can it be that some schools match in the single digit? If some schools have match rate in the 80%, one could reasonably extrapolate that some schools will have very low match numbers. This is important for the students applying—why do you want to go to a school that cannot offer you some degree of hope that after four years you will obtain a residency?

What are the reasons for such low match rate? It is a multifactorial issue. We have already mentioned some factors in a previous section. The reasons for low matches includes the following:

- Lower Step 1 and Step scoresYes, there will be large number of very good students with great scores above 220. But will be also a number with scores below 200. We know, from all available data, that those with low scores will have problems obtaining interviews and matching. Some programs do not interview students with Step 1 scores below 205.
- A degree of bias from program directors that will accept an average US graduate above a very good Caribbean graduate, and there are some who will not take a foreign graduate.
- Inconsistent advising. Graduates applying to hospitals where they have low chances.
- The very large pool of international medical graduates makes a fair and just selection difficult.

In brief, the match is not a precise, scientific process. It is influenced by the opinions and biases of program directors, the competitiveness of the program and the specialty. The applicant's performance in an interview and his scores and grades are also important factors as well.

The process is a distorted meritocracy.

Match results for Caribbean students will get better when their scores get higher in NBME examinations and the schools provide their students proper advice offered by people with experience in resident selection. Is there bias in selection? I know of some. There is also some literature to suggest, but I have found no real statistical proof. That feeling will dissipate when the examination scores of Caribbean graduates equals or exceeds those of US graduates.

The enclosed table contains good information, and it gives some idea what the probabilities of students according to Step 2 scores. This table was published in a previous page but it is important to repeat it.

Table 17-4

	Matched		**Not Matched**	
Step 2 Scores	**US Grads**	**US IMG**	**US Grads**	**US IMG**
Anesthesiology	241	238	223	212
Emer. Medicine	243	235	225	223
Family Medicine	234	213	216	203
Internal Med.	243	228	219	210
Neurology	241	222	236	206
Ob-Gyn	242	232	225	213
Pathology	241	226	236	206
Pediatrics	241	224	219	208
Phys. Med. & Rehab	234	231	220	212
Psychiatry	233	211	216	202
Radiology	249	241	236	223
Surgery- General	245	234	226	216

All available information suggests that the match is indeed more competitive for the graduates of several Caribbean schools, especially the newer schools or those without an established

reputation. We base this statement and the following comments on 2016 NRMP data.

- US graduates with the right scores will continue to be preferred over any international graduate with a similar score. If we assume that 93.8% of US graduates matched, they will occupy 17,057 of the 27,860 available positions.
- This leaves 10,803 positions for all remaining applicants. Another 2339 positions will be taken by DO graduates, who have a match rate of 80%.
- Applying to the match are 5,323 US citizens from international schools, and in the last five years, this number has grown by 23%.
- That leaves 12,805 applicants for the remaining 8,464 positions, a total of 1.5 applicants per position. If the match statements of the more recognized Caribbean schools are correct (For example, according to Bloomberg.com/news/2013, 76% of Ross students and 79% of American University of the Caribbean secured residency positions through the NRMP). If this will continue, it will erode another 1,700 positions from the remaining pool.

  This would then suggest that the remaining 5,700 positions will be disputed by US citizens graduated of lesser-known foreign schools, foreign citizens, graduates of foreign schools, and the few US graduates applying to the match a second time. That tells us that for this subgroup there will be two applicants per position. Yes, these are suppositions, but they are based on some available hard data and decades of experience.
- The match data for all US international graduates has remained quite stable around 52%. If the number of graduates from the most recognized schools remain the same or increase, it should be a clear message to newer or less reputable Caribbean schools. Many of their students will be heavy in debt with an MD degree but lmited access to a residency and no way to become a practicing physician in the United States.
- The NRMP data must also be examined by specialty to determine the likelihood that an international graduate secures

position in the specialty. Using the 2016 NRMP report, we can observe that the following specialties selected only graduates of US schools in their match.

Dermatology
Medicine-Anesthesia
Medicine-Dermatology
Interventional Radiology
Pediatrics-Emergency Medicine
Psychiatry-Neurology

- At the other end of the spectrum, some specialties have the lowest percentage of US graduates matched, and these include the following:

  Family Medicine (45% of US Graduates)
  Medicine-Preventive Medicine (42.9%)
  Internal Medicine (Categorical) (46.9%)
  Pathology (42.%)
  Surgery-Preliminary PG1 (39%)
  Pediatrics-Primary (43%)
  Neurology (53%)
- The above percentages may be able to provide a partial explanation as to why Caribbean graduates tend to apply to primary care specialties. They have a greater probability of matching.

There are some other points that need to be emphasized.

- PG1 positions have increased by 16%, while the number of Caribbean students in the match has increased by 21%. What is the point of increasing or maintaining class size if, at the end of four years, the number of residencies does not increase sufficiently?
- In five years, the number of US students has increased by 9%. With time we will see that the number of US graduates will increase even further as a result of new schools and increased enrollment. If the preference for US graduates does not change,

the match for Caribbean students will be even more competitive for everyone.

Advise to applicants: be sure, before you accept going to a school, that you know it has a record of high probabilities to obtain a residency. Without one all your effort will be of little use.

- The NRMP results demonstrate a distinct preference, as expected, for US graduates and a high match rate for DOs. There are little changes from year to year for graduates of Caribbean schools.

In conclusion,

- the NRMP data for Caribbean medical students suggests that their success is quite comparable to all international graduates and definitively lower than graduates of DO schools;
- the issue of Caribbean schools graduates unable to obtain a residency is of critical importance since it leaves a number of people with a degree that they cannot put to practical use and have large loans to repay;
- the continued increase in enrollment in US schools both allopathic and osteopathic, associated with an increase of enrollment in Caribbean schools will be met by a limited number of clinical training sites and graduate medical education positions. This is clearly detailed in a recent AAMC Publication.

CHAPTER 20

Some Final Thoughts

1. The very good Caribbean medical schools are here to stay. I come to this conclusion for several reasons.
    - It will be a long time before the capacity of US medical schools can accommodate the demand.
    - Some Caribbean schools are expanding their marketing efforts and starting to attract an international student body.
    - Some schools have received major financial investments from foreign sources.
    - Ownership of the schools has expanded and includes foreign investors.
2. The US applicant pool has limited elasticity and will cease to grow soon. There may be some growth from foreign student applicants. Caribbean medical schools will need to review their marketing strategies, curriculum and teaching methords to accommodate the changes in student population
3. The growth of new medical and DO schools increases the competition. A bottleneck will develop for clinical training. Caribbean schools should either get new clinical training sites or adjust class size to clinical training resources.
4. As the competition for new student increases, a natural selection among Caribbean schools will take place. The rules of the market will apply, and some of the weaker schools will close unless they concentrate on the foreign market or improve quality and outcomes
5. The new regulations regarding accreditation that will go into effect in 2023 will put pressure on smaller and less-funded schools that will have to do a lot of work to meet the new accreditation standards.

6. New accreditation requirements likely to increase cost and decrease profit margin. Some schools cannot continue to increase tuition.
7. The more expensive schools will not be able to sustain their profit margins, and they will have to lower the tuition. All medical schools will have to learn to accept a reduction in revenues and a reasonable profit margin or cease to exist.
8. If available capital exists, some of the newer schools will improve quality and reputation. When that happens, price competition will start. There are already big differences in tuition between schools. Some schools are charging tuition comparable to 14. US schools. Once the quality and, hence, reputation and market position of the newer schools increases, when their licensing examination results is competitive with older, more respected" schools, and the placement of graduates in residencies also improves. These schools will compete with the better-positioned schools.
9. For decades Caribbean schools have worked independently, in competition with each other. It is time they create an association with selective membership criteria. This association will represent them in front of government organizations and legislators, serve as their lobbyist, and also be the repository of accurate, validated data.
10. After this many years of benign neglect and disdainful disrespect, the AAMC should recognize that Caribbean schools are here to stay and some have reached educational outcomes comparable to many US schools. There are multiple ways for coexistence and cooperation. They should create some agreements beneficial to all.
11. One suggestion is that AAMC invites some Caribbean schools to become associate members of the organization. The selection of the schools should be determined on quality of education, graduation rates, licensing examination average scores, and NRMP match rates, facilities and other salient factors.
12. A second option would be for Caribbean schools to set up their own professional organization, but I believe a single organization would give bigger lobbying power and serve as the only data repository for schools that serve primarily American students.

13. Once the first step is taken by the AAMC, US medical schools should try to form a working relationship with the good and recognized schools. How can that be done? US veterinarian schools have done it. They have made agreements with Caribbean private veterinarian schools to provide the clinical training for their students and get paid for it. Students do all the basic sciences in a Caribbean island, and the clinical training in a US veterinary school, graduating with degrees from the Caribbean school. By creating similar relationships and accepting very good students who have completed basic sciences in the Caribbean (and passing NBME step 1), medical schools could increase revenues and decrease overhead.

US schools should expand class size to meet the demand. They may want to look at the Caribbean model, including the following:

- Take more risks in admitting new students with weaker academic records.
- Create preparatory courses to bring these students to a competitive level. These preparatory courses have been very successful and have allowed students with borderline credentials to complete basic sciences and pass licensing examinations. We are aware of at least one US school that has a comparable program.

  Have two classes a year. The issue of faculty not being able to teach twice a year should not be a real issue. The issue of clinical training sites has many potential solutions once that US schools begin to pay hospitals an adequate amount 16. US and Caribbean schools are in competition for clinical training sites. Hospitals and clinics are having financial issues and benefit from the revenue provided by Caribbean schools for allowing their students to train. As of this moment, payments have reached up to $500 per student per weak. Many US schools do not pay hospitals or teaching faculty. US schools need to accept that having students creates costs that may not be fully recovered. Compensating hospitals, clinics and physicians could give schools leverage and open new teaching sites.

Perhaps they will have to compete with Caribbean schools, and competition is good and it may result in some working relationships.

17. US schools may benefit by working with some Caribbean schools and create international experiences so popular with medical students.
18. Research opportunities could develop between the medical schools and perhaps their school of Public Health. Some examples for research initiatives are the following:
    - Diabetes and hypertension research
    - Cross cultural research
    - Tropical medicine research
    - Mental health research
    - Clinical trials
    - Health system research or model comparison
    - Multiple education research issues

    An additional comment regarding student financial aid. The money flowing to Caribbean schools cannot be looked only as tuition help for medical students or a way to ensure the profit margin of some investor. It must also be looked as part of US foreign aid to underdeveloped Caribbean countries. This money creates jobs and increases commerce. These funds contribute significantly to raise the GDP of these small countries. The fact is that the private sector makes a great contribution to developing countries. For example, DeVry offers tuition benefits for undergraduate and graduate degrees for its local staff in Dominica, Saint Kitts, and Sint Maarten. That has allowed local staff to obtain college or graduate school degrees otherwise unavailable in their country.

In Conclusion

Many Caribbean medical schools have evolved, grown, and improved since their origin, and they offer today good and viable alternatives to those students who failed to get admission to a US medical schools.

Unfortunately, several schools still operate, and their poor results tarnish the image of those that have tried very hard to offer an education that compares to American schools.

If American organized medicine offers a hand to those good schools, creating good cooperative arrangements, everyone's educational results will continue to improve and the number of good graduates will grow. This will help address the much discussed issue of physician shortage.

APPENDIX 1

Process for Recognition of Medical School Accrediting Agencies

THE FOLLOWING IS information pertinent to accreditation, applicable to all medical schools in the Caribbean region as published by the ECFMG

February 13, 2015
Process for Recognition of Medical School Accrediting Agencies Now Available

Accrediting agencies are encouraged to apply now to prepare for ECFMG's 2023 accreditation requirement In September 2010, ECFMG announced that, effective in 2023, physicians applying for ECFMG Certification will be required to graduate from a medical school that has been appropriately accredited.

Since that announcement, a process for recognizing the agencies that accredit medical schools has been developed. This process will allow medical schools accredited by recognized agencies, and their graduates, to meet ECFMG's accreditation requirement.

As announced in ECFMG's March 2013 update, the World Federation for Medical Education (WFME), in collaboration with the Foundation for Advancement of International Medical Education and Research (FAIMER®), has developed a Programme for Recognition of Accrediting Agencies. This Programme is the culmination of a pilot launched in 2011 by

WFME and FAIMER to develop a meaningful process for evaluating and recognizing accrediting agencies using globally accepted criteria.

Detailed information, including an explanation of the process and the required application forms, is available at the WFME website at http://wfme.org/accreditation/accrediting-accreditors. Since WFME's Programme became available, several accrediting agencies have applied for and been granted recognition by WFME through this process. These agencies include:

- Association for Evaluation and Accreditation of Medical Education Programs (Turkey)
- Caribbean Accreditation Authority for Education in Medicine and other Health Professions (CAAMHP)
- Liaison Committee on Medical Education (LCME, USA) and the
- Committee on Accreditation of Canadian Medical Schools (CACMS)

For more information on agencies recognized by WFME, refer to the WFME website at http://wfme.org/accreditation/accrediting-accreditors/recognition-process/87-8-recognition-ofaccreditation-agencies-agencies-that-are-recognised/file.

With the 2023 effective date approaching, ECFMG encourages all agencies that accredit medical schools to visit the WFME website, review the available information, and take action to allow medical schools and their graduates to be in compliance by the deadline. Questions regarding WFME's recognition process may be e-mailed to WFME at accreditation@wfme.org.

Accrediting agencies, medical schools, and international medical graduates should monitor the ECFMG website at www.ecfmg.org/accreditation for updates.

APPENDIX 2

34 CFR 600.55 - Additional criteria for determining whether a foreign graduate medical school is eligible to apply to participate in the Direct Loan Program.

(a) General.

(1) The Secretary considers a foreign graduate medical school to be eligible to apply to participate in the title IV, HEA programs if, in addition to satisfying the criteria of this part (except the criterion in §600.54 that the institution be public or private nonprofit), the school satisfies the criteria of this section.

(2) A foreign graduate medical school must provide, and in the normal course require its students to complete, a program of clinical training and classroom medical instruction of not less than 32 months in length, that is supervised closely by members of the school's faculty and that—

(i) Is provided in facilities adequately equipped and staffed to afford students comprehensive clinical training and classroom medical instruction;

(ii) Is approved by all medical licensing boards and evaluating bodies whose views are considered relevant by the Secretary; and

(iii) As part of its clinical training, does not offer more than two electives consisting of no more than eight weeks per student at a site located in a foreign country other than the country in which the main campus is located or in the United States, unless that location is included in the accreditation of a medical program accredited by the Liaison Committee on Medical Education (LCME) or the American Osteopathic Association (AOA).

(3) A foreign graduate medical school must appoint for the program described in paragraph (a)(2) of this section only those faculty members whose academic credentials are the equivalent of credentials required of faculty members teaching the same or similar courses at medical schools in the United States.

(4) A foreign graduate medical school must have graduated classes during each of the two twelve-month periods immediately preceding the date the Secretary receives the school's request for an eligibility determination.

(b) **Accreditation.** A foreign graduate medical school must—

(1) Be approved by an accrediting body—

(i) That is legally authorized to evaluate the quality of graduate medical school educational programs and facilities in the country where the school is located; and

(ii) Whose standards of accreditation of graduate medical schools have been evaluated by the NCFMEA or its successor committee of medical experts and have been determined to be comparable to standards of accreditation applied to medical schools in the United States; or

(2) Be a public or private nonprofit educational institution that satisfies the requirements in§600.4(a)(5)(i).

(c) **Admission criteria.**

(1) A foreign graduate medical school having a post-baccalaureate/ equivalent medical program must require students accepted for admission who are US citizens, nationals, or permanent residents to have taken the Medical College Admission Test (MCAT) and to have reported their scores to the foreign graduate medical school; and

(2) A foreign graduate medical school must determine the consent requirements for, and require the necessary consents of, all students accepted for admission for whom the school must report to enable the school to comply with the collection and submission requirements of paragraph (d) of this section.

(d) Collection and submission of data.

(1) A foreign graduate medical school must obtain, at its own expense, and submit, by the date required by paragraph (d)(3) of this section—

(i) To its accrediting authority and, on request, to the Secretary, the scores on the MCAT or successor examination, of all students admitted during the preceding calendar year who are US citizens, nationals, or eligible permanent residents, together with a statement of the number of times each student took the examination;

(ii) To its accrediting authority and, on request, to the Secretary, the percentage of students graduating during the preceding calendar year (including at least all graduates who are US citizens, nationals, or eligible permanent residents) who obtain placement in an accredited US medical residency program;

(iii) To the Secretary, except as provided for in paragraph (d)(2) of this section, all scores, disaggregated by step/test—i.e., Step 1, Step 2—Clinical Skills (Step 2-CS), and Step 2—Clinical Knowledge (Step 2-CK), or the successor examinations—and attempt, earned during the preceding calendar year by each student and graduate, on Step 1, Step 2-CS, and Step 2-CK, or the successor examinations, of the US Medical Licensing Examination (USMLE), together with the dates the student has taken each test, including any failed tests;

(iv) To the Secretary, a statement of its citizenship rate for the preceding calendar year for a school that is subject to paragraph (f)(1)(i)(A) of this section, together with a description of the methodology used in deriving the rate that is acceptable to the Secretary.

(2) In lieu of submitting the information required in paragraph (d)(1)(iii) of this section to the Secretary, a foreign graduate medical school that is not subject to paragraph (f)(4) of this section may agree to allow the Educational Commission for Foreign Medical Graduates (ECFMG) or other responsible third party to calculate the rate described in paragraph (f)(1)(ii) and (f)(3) of this section for the preceding calendar year and provide the rate directly to the

Secretary on the school's behalf with a copy to the foreign graduate medical school, provided—

(i) The foreign graduate medical school has provided by April 30 to the Secretary written consent acceptable to the Secretary to reliance by the Secretary on the pass rate as calculated by the ECFMG or other responsible third party for purposes of determining compliance with paragraph (f)(1)(ii) and (f)(3) of this section for the preceding calendar year; and

(ii) The foreign graduate medical school agrees in its written consent that for the preceding calendar year the rate as calculated by the ECFMG or other designated third party will be conclusive for purposes of determining compliance with paragraph (f)(1)(ii) and (f)(3) of this section.

(3) A foreign graduate medical school must submit the data it collects in accordance with paragraph (d)(1) of this section no later than April 30 of each year, unless the Secretary specifies a different date through a notice in the Federal Register.

(e) Requirements for clinical training.

(1)

(i) A foreign graduate medical school must have—

(A) A formal affiliation agreement with any hospital or clinic at which all or a portion of the school's core clinical training or required clinical rotations are provided; and

(B) Either a formal affiliation agreement or other written arrangements with any hospital or clinic at which all or a portion of its clinical rotations that are not required are provided, except for those locations that are not used regularly, but instead are chosen by individual students who take no more than two electives at the location for no more than a total of eight weeks.

(ii) The agreements described in paragraph (e)(1)(i) of this section must state how the following will be addressed at each site—

(A) Maintenance of the school's standards;

(B) Appointment of faculty to the medical school staff;

(C) Design of the curriculum;

(D) Supervision of students;

(E) Evaluation of student performance; and

(F) Provision of liability insurance.

(2) A foreign graduate medical school must notify its accrediting body within one year of any material changes in—

(i) The educational programs, including changes in clinical training programs; and

(ii) The overseeing bodies and in the formal affiliation agreements with hospitals and clinics described in paragraph (e)(1)(i) of this section.

(f) **Citizenship and USMLE pass rate percentages.**

(1)

(i) During the calendar year preceding the year for which any of the school's students seeks an title IV, HEA program loan, at least 60 percent of those enrolled as full-time regular students in the school and at least 60 percent of the school's most recent graduating class must have been persons who did not meet the citizenship and residency criteria contained in section 484(a)(5) of the HEA, 20 USC. 1091(a)(5); or

(A) The school must have had a clinical training program approved by a State prior to January 1, 2008, and must continue to operate a clinical training program in at least one State that approves the program; and

(ii) Except as provided in paragraph (f)(4) of this section, for a foreign graduate medical school outside of Canada, for Step 1, Step 2-CS, and Step 2-CK, or the successor examinations, of the USMLE administered by the ECFMG, at least 75 percent of the school's students and graduates who took that step/test of the examination in the year preceding the year for which any of the school's students seeks a title IV, HEA program loan must have received a passing score on that step/test and are taking the step/test for the first time; or

(2)

(i) The school must have had a clinical training program approved by a State as of January 1, 1992; and

(ii) The school must continue to operate a clinical training program in at least one State that approves the program.

(3) In performing the calculation required in paragraph (f)(1)(ii) of this section, a foreign graduate medical school shall—

(i) Include as a graduate each student who graduated from the school during the three years preceding the year for which the calculation is performed and who took that step/test for the first time in that year; and

(ii) Include students and graduates who take more than one step/test of the USMLE examination for the first time in the same year in the denominator for each of those steps/tests;

(4)

(i) If the calculation described in paragraph (f)(1)(ii) of this section would result in any step/test pass rate based on fewer than eight students, a single pass rate for the school is determined instead based on the performance of the school's students and graduates on Step 1, Step 2-CS, and Step 2-CK combined;

(ii) If combining the results on all three step/tests as permitted in paragraph (f)(4)(i) of this section would result in a pass rate based on fewer than eight step/test results, the school is deemed to have no pass rate for that year and the results for the year are combined with each subsequent year until a pass rate based on at least eight step/test results is derived.

(g) Other criteria.

(1) As part of establishing, publishing, and applying reasonable satisfactory academic progress standards, a foreign graduate medical school must include as a quantitative component a maximum timeframe in which a student must complete his or her educational program that must—

(i) Be no longer than 150 percent of the published length of the educational program measured in academic years, terms, credit hours attempted, clock hours completed, etc., as appropriate; and

(ii) Meet the requirements of §668.16(e)(2)(ii)(B), (C) and (D).

(2) (A foreign graduate medical school must document the educational remediation it provides to assist students in making satisfactory academic progress.

(3) A foreign graduate medical school must publish all the languages in which instruction is offered.

(h) **Location of a program.**

(1) Except as provided in paragraph (h)(3)(ii) of this section, all portions of a graduate medical education program offered to US students must be located in a country whose medical school accrediting standards are comparable to standards used in the United States, as determined by the NCFMEA, except for clinical training sites located in the United States.

(2) No portion of the graduate medical educational program offered to US students, other than the clinical training portion of the program, may be located outside of the country in which the main campus of the foreign graduate medical school is located.

(3)

(i) Except as provided in paragraph (h)(3)(ii) of this section, for any part of the clinical training portion of the educational program located in a foreign country other than the country in which the main campus is located or in the United States, in order for students attending the site to be eligible to borrow title IV, HEA program funds—

(A) The site must be located in an NCFMEA approved comparable foreign country;

(B) The institution's medical accrediting agency must have conducted an on-site evaluation and specifically approved the clinical training site; and

(C) Clinical instruction must be offered in conjunction with medical educational programs offered to students enrolled in accredited medical schools located in that approved foreign country.

(ii) A clinical training site located in a foreign country other than the country in which the main campus is located or in the United States is not required to meet the requirements of paragraph (h)(3)(i) of this section in order for students attending that site to be eligible to borrow title IV, HEA program funds if—

(A) The location is included in the accreditation of a medical program accredited by the Liaison Committee on Medical Education (LCME) or the American Osteopathic Association (AOA); or

(B) No individual student takes more than two electives at the location and the combined length of the electives does not exceed eight weeks.

APPENDIX 3

ENCLOSED IS SOME very basic information about the schools as provided by each school website, or in some cases by l information and shared by faculty and graduates. They will be presented in alphabetic order.

All American Institute of Medical Sciences www.aaims.edu.jm)

All American Institute of Medical Science is located in Jamaica and began operations in 2009. It was chartered by the Government of Jamaica in 2011, and provisionally accredited by the Caribbean Accreditation Authority for Education in Medicine and other Health Professions (CAAM-HP) in 2010 with an annual renewal to 2015.The university began classes in 2011 at its Jamaica campus and graduated its first class in 2014.

American University of Antigua (www.auamed.org)

Established in 2004, the school was developed by Neil Simon, Esq., former president of Ross University.

In 2008, Manipal Education and Medical Group purchased the college from New York–based Greater Caribbean Learning Resources Inc. and formed Maniple Education Americas, LLC. The school is currently owned by the Manipal Group that, in addition to the school in Antigua, has schools and colleges in India, Malaysia and Dubai.

In January 2010, AUA opened its seventeen-acre (69,000 m^2) campus. The \$60 million facility houses more than 75,000 square feet (7,000 m^2) of classrooms, a simulation lab, a multistory library, study rooms, an amphitheater, a courtyard, a gym, tennis courts, and administrative and faculty offices.

The school has continued to grow and its students are now eligible to receive US financial aid. This school demonstrates something that was discussed, namely the entry into Caribbean education of non-American investors who likely see potential to expand the student body with students coming from different countries.

AUA has received accreditation from New York and California and from CAAM-HP.

AUA has signed an affiliation agreement with the Florida International University Herbert Wertheim College of Medicine that allows AUA clinical students to complete all of their core clinical rotations in the Greater Miami Area.

l Medical U (www.aimu.us)

American International Medical University, located in Saint Lucia, is an independent affiliate of AIM-U International Group and is affiliated with Washington Adventist hospital, Takoma Park, Maryland. The school is listed in the FAIMER International Medical Education Directory (IMED) effective in 2007 and in the World Health Organization's World Directory of Medical Schools.

There is no information available on graduates or residency placements.

Information from 2015 describes substantial legal issues as reported by local newspapers and radios,.

American University of Barbados (www.aubmed.org)

American University of Barbados of Medicine (AUB) was founded in 2011 and chartered by the Government of Barbados. It is listed in WHO list of medical schools and in the International Medical School Directory (IMED)

American University of Saint Vincent (www.ausmed.us)

It is listed in the WHO list of medical schools and in the International Medical School Directory (IMED)

In February 2016 it enrolled a new class of twenty-eight students. There is no information on graduates.

American University of the Caribbean (www.aucmed/edu)

Founded by American educator Dr. Paul Tien in 1978, the main campus of the American University of the Caribbean was originally located on the island of Montserrat. The story of AUC is one of determination!

While a medical campus was being constructed on Montserrat, AUC started conducting classes in a rented space on the campus of the College of Mount Saint Joseph in Cincinnati, Ohio. The first class, with 107 students, started on August 14, 1978.

The government of Montserrat granted AUC a twenty-five-acre parcel of land where a new campus was built. AUC began conducting classes at its new campus in Montserrat in January 1980.

On September 17, 1989, Hurricane Hugo hit the island, severely damaging the campus. Students and faculty were evacuated. While the Montserrat campus was being rebuilt, AUC operated at a temporary location in Plainview, Texas, where classes started again on October 17, 1989.

The Montserrat campus was rebuilt and AUC reopened it for classes in September 1990.

The Soufriere volcano erupted on July 18, 1995, rendering much of the island uninhabitable and its population evacuated. Students and faculty were evacuated. The campus was buried under volcanic ash.

In September 1995, 250 students were sent to a temporary location in Belize, and 280 students were sent to a temporary location in Sint Maarten.

On September 5, 1995, Hurricane Luis hit Sint Maarten, destroyed much of its infrastructure, and delayed the opening of the Sint Maarten operation by three weeks.

AUC finally settled in Sint Marten and gradually gained recognition for its medical education.

AUC purchased a parcel of land in Sint Martin and construction of a permanent campus began in July 1996. The new campus opened on May 1, 1998. The school grew and gained very good reputation.

AUC is listed with the World Health Organization's Avicenna directory and in the ECFMG IMED/FAIMER database of medical schools, is accredited by the Accreditation Commission of Colleges of Medicine and by the states of California, New York, and Florida and is approved for US financial aid.

In 2013 AUC was purchased by DeVry University for $210 million.

American University of Integrative Services (www.auis.edu)

Located in Sint Maarten School and was previously known as the University of Saint Eustatius School of Medicine.

It began instruction on September 1, 1999. Subsequently, the university was awarded a charter by the governor of Saint Eustatius on April 21. The school, under the new ownership and management of Georgia-based International Educational Management Resources, set up new administration and operations on the Caribbean island of Saint Maarten in September 2013, and changed its name to American University of Integrated Sciences, Saint Maarten School of Medicine. Its curriculum incorporated the teaching of alternative medicine practices into its existing US curriculum–based programs.

The university is listed in FAIMER International Medical Education Directory(IMED) and in the Avicenna Directory for medicine.

Atlantic University School of Medicine (www.ausom.edu.lc)

he school's application was approved by the cabinet of Saint Lucia in 2010. It is listed in the FAIMER International Medical Education Directory (IMED) effective in 2010 and in the World Health Organization's World Directory of Medical Schools. It is not accredited by the Caribbean Accreditation Authority for Education in Medicine and other Health Professions (CAAM-HP) as of 2015.

There is little, if any information regarding school, academic programs, or graduates.

Avalon University School of Medicine (www.avalonu.org)

AUSOM was founded in 2003 in Bonaire in the Netherlands Antilles) as the Xavier University School of Medicine. In 2010, the university relocated to Curacao and changed its name to Avalon University School of Medicine.

It is chartered by the Ministry of Education of Curacao to offer an MD degree and listed in the FAIMER International Medical Education Directory (IMED) and in the Avicenna Directory for medicine. AUSOM has also submitted a request for accreditation by the Caribbean Accreditation Authority for Education in Medicine and other Health Professions. As of August 7, 2015, Avalon University School of Medicine is not approved by the CAAM-HP.

In 2016 Avalon has posted a listing of residency matches in United States and Canada that includes seventy-six graduates.

Aureus University School of Medicine (www.aureusuniversity.com)

Aureus University School of Medicine was founded in 2004 in Aruba. On January 4, 2011, the school announced it was changing its name from All Saints University of Medicine to coincide with facility enhancements and to distinguish itself from universities with the same name. The current campus was completed in 2006 and contains a medical library, laboratories, student recreation center, and twelve lecture rooms.

Aureus University School of Medicine is chartered in and recognized by the government of Aruba. andis listed in the FAIMER International Medical Education Directory and in the Avicenna Directory for medicine.

The school graduated fifteen students in 2015 and sixteen in 2016.

Caribbean Medical University (www.cmued.org)

It is located in Curacao and was founded in 2007. CMU has an average class of twenty-seven students. It was chartered in and recognized by the government of the Netherlands Antilles on November 9, 2007, and is listed in the FAIMER International Medical Education Directory and in the Avicenna Directory for medicine.

No additional information is available regarding students or graduates.

Central America Health Sciences University (Belize, www.cahsu.edu)

Located in Belize City, Belize, it was founded in 1996 It is chartered by the Government of Belize and is approved by the Ministry of Education in Belize. It is listed in the World Directory of Medical Schools and is recognized by the Educational Commission on Foreign Medical Graduates (ECFMG). It is also recognized by the General Medical Council (GMC) of the United Kingdom.

College of Medicine and Health Sciences (www.comhssl.net)

COMHS is located in Saint Lucia, combining traditional education and distance education Once known as Destiny University, COMHS indicates that it is a cost-effective opportunity for students worldwide to become physicians. Students can access courses anywhere in the world to study, complete assignments, or take exams using Skype or E-learning. Students can also attend classes, full time.

No information regarding graduates or residency placements is available.

Georgetown American University (www.gau.edu.gy)

No information on the history of the institution or specific data on class size.

International American University College of Medicine (www.iau.edu.lc)

Located in Saint Lucia and granted a trade license for offshore schools. It should be noted that there is no governmental licensing or regulation of offshore medical schools for this or any other medical school operating in the country.

The school is listed in both FAIMERs and the World Directory of medical schools. It has obtained approval from the Government of Canada and its application is pending before the CAAM-HP

Ross University (www.rossu.edu)

It was founded by Robert Ross, a New York entrepreneur. In 1976, when a staff member's son who had been studying medicine in the Dominican Republic was rejected by the American hospitals for clerkships. Mr. Ross started a business helping students from foreign medical schools get accepted at hospitals in the United States. Ross University School of Medicine started in 1978, financed by Mr. Ross's investment of $15–$20 million. There were eleven students, and classes were held in a hotel.

He offered a program that was more accelerated and less expensive than those offered by most medical schools. Initially it was castigated by the American Medical Association as substandard, but he obtained approval for students to qualify for federal student loans.

Graduates had to pass the same tests as graduates of American schools, and many accepted hard-to-fill positions in primary care, often in run-down urban neighborhoods. "They are a godsend," a Brooklyn hospital administrator told Forbes in 1983.

In 2000, Mr. Ross sold the medical school, along with a veterinary school he started on Saint Kitts in 1980, for about $135 million to an investment group. This investment group appointed Mr. T. Foster as president, and a number of changes were implemented, such as requiring an MCAT score to apply, implementing the National Board of Medical Examiners Comprehensive at the end of Basic Sciences and dictating that students should pass the Comp before being certified to take Step 1. Students were given three chances to pass the Comp, and if they failed to do so, they were dismissed from medical school. As a result, the quality of students and of graduates improved, and so did the reputation of the school.

Major improvements in technology and facilities were put in place. New classrooms' construction expanded aging facilities.

In 1983, this investment group sold Ross University to DeVry for $320 million. DeVry has continued to build new facilities and classrooms, including a state-of-the-art simulation center, a new student center with small meeting rooms as well as new eating facilities and indoor and outdoor athletic facilities.

At present, Ross is one of the premier medical schools in the Caribbean.

Ross University

Saba University (www.saba.edu)

Saba University is located in Saba, Dutch island and is a legally recognized entity of higher education in the Netherlands. The school is accredited by the NVAO (in Dutch, Nederlands-Vlaamse Accreditatieorganisatie), the Accreditation Organization of the Netherlands and Flanders. And also by New York, California, and Florida.

Saba University School of Medicine graduates are eligible to practice medicine in Canada, Puerto Rico, and all fifty US states.

Saint Martinus (www.martinus.edu)

Established as Saint Martinus University on May 22, 2000. In October 2005, the school had half the number of students it needed to break even, and in October 2007, Banco de Caribe announced an auction of the university property. The education of students never halted and the auction never actually manifested.

Saint Martinus University was chartered by the Government of the Netherlands Antilles in 2001 and recognized by the Curacao Ministry of Health in 2005. It is listed in the FAIMER International Medical Education Directory (IMED) and in the Avicenna Directory for medicine. Is not approved by the CAAM-HP.

Saint Matthews (www.ctmattewns.edu)

SMU was founded in Belize in 1997 by Jeffrey S. Sersland. In 2002, the school moved to the Cayman Islands. The School of Veterinary Medicine was established in 2005.The school was acquired in 2005 by Equinox Capital in conjunction with Chicago-based Prairie Capital.

SMU is chartered by the government of the Cayman Islands and is accredited by the Accreditation Commission of Colleges of Medicine. The school is also accredited by the New York State Department of Education (NYSED) and the Florida Department of Education's Commission for Independent Education for the purpose of providing clinical rotations in those states and is listed in the FAIMER International Medical Education Directory and in the Avicenna Directory for medicine.

Saint George's University (www.sgu.edu)

On July 23, 1976, the founders, Charles Modica, Louis Modica, Edward McGowan, and Patrick F. Adams obtained an act from the Grenada's Parliament establishing St. George's University School of Medicine.

With a handful of students and faculty, classes at St. George's School of Medicine began on January 17, 1977. The University has continued to grow and today it has over 6,000 students studying in 48 academic degree programs, including an MD as wells as a veterinary program and stand-alone dual-degree graduate programs that include MBA and an accredited MPH program. Clinical programs are offered in the United States and the UK.

It is now one of the ranking schools in the Caribbean and it has graduated over 10,000 physicians practicing in the United States. It is recognized in all 50 states where its graduates con obtain a license.

A class room at St George's School of Medicine.

Saint James University (www.sjsm.org)

Saint James School of Medicine was established in Bonaire in 1999 and began instruction in 2000. In 2011, it opened a second campus in Anguilla and, in 2014, opened a third Caribbean medical school campus in Saint Vincent and the Grenadines and Anguilla. The school was founded in 2001, and have a current enrollment of around 1,000 students.

Saint James School of Medicine is recognized by the Medical Council for Canada by FAIMER and ECFMG.

Spartan University (www.spartanedu.org)

Spartan was established in Saint Lucia on January 7, 1980. It started as Saint Lucia Health Sciences University. In November 1983, the school was renamed Spartan Health Sciences University. A school of veterinary medicine was opened on January 14, 2015, and was developed in collaboration with Techmedics Inc.

The school indicates that it has received provisional accreditation from CAAM-HP. The medical boards of California, Indiana, and North Dakota have listed Spartan as an institution whose graduates are ineligible for licensure.

Texila American University (www.tauedu.prg)

Texila American University is owned by the Texila American University Limited – Hong Kong (TAU-HK). TAU-HK is a project of the ALLTERE Education Management Company. The university is located in Guyana, and offers undergraduate and postgraduate degrees in medicine, nursing, public health and allied sciences.[2]

The school is registered with the National Accreditation Council of Guyana. It is listed in both FAIMERs and the World Directory of Medical Schools.

Trinity School of Medicine (www.trinityschoolofmedicine.org)

This school is located in Saint Vincent and the Grenadines. It opened in 2008. The Trinity School of Medicine was chartered and licensed in Saint Vincent and the Grenadines on 11 April 2008 and listed in the FAIMER International Medical Education Directory (IMED) effective on 19 September 2008. In July 2015, Trinity School of Medicine also received CAAM-HP accreditation.

University of Science, Arts and Technology (www.usat.edu)

Located in Montserrat, the university opened in 2003. Though the school is listed by the Foundation for Advancement of International Medical Education and Research, accreditation has been denied by the CAAM-HP in both 2007 and 2012.

University of Health Science (Saint Kitts, www.umhs.sk.org)

When DeVry completed the purchase of Ross University, it established a noncompete agreement that prevented Robert Ross to establish a medical school for a prescribed period. The agreement also precluded the use of the name Ross for any future new school. This was legally argued, and DeVry prevailed.

The legal case did not deter Robert Ross. He proceeded to open a nursing school in Saint Kitts with high quality facilities. Obvious to all was that, when legally feasible, he would open a medical school. This happened in 2008 under the leadership of Warren Ross, Dr. Ross's son, who had been very involved in the management of Ross University before. He had the knowledge and business expertise to quickly start a good operation. He has indeed succeeded.

Warren Ross had some specific goals. He wanted a modern facility, a traditional curriculum, and a moderate tuition. He had the proper contact to recruit and also to establish clinical sites in the United States. UMHS indicates a Step 1 passing of 93% and good placements for the first graduating classes.

The school has built modern facilities and added excellent technology. Its reputation is growing with time and its graduates placing in residencies.

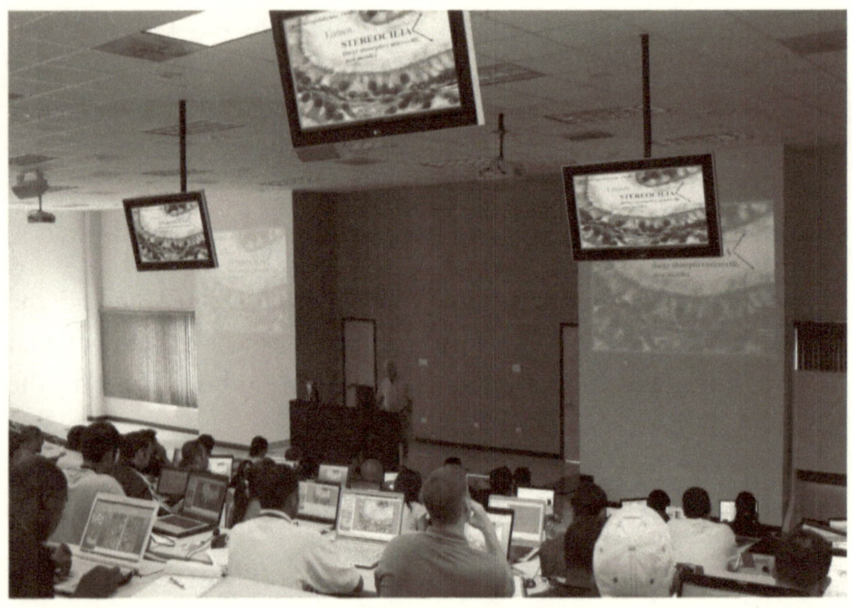

University of Health Sciences (Antigua, www.uhsa.ag)

UHSA was established in 1982 and began instruction in 1983. UHSA is recognized by the Government of Antigua and Barbuda. Because of this recognition, the university is listed in the FAIMER International Medical Education Directory (IMED). It is also listed in the Avicenna Directory for medicine.

The medical board of California, Indiana, Kansas, and North Dakota has listed UHSA as an institution whose graduates are not eligible for licensure in the state.

Windsor University (www.windsor.edu)

Windsor was founded in December 1998 on Grand Turk Island in Turks and Caicos. Instruction began with a class of eight students. In 2000, the university relocated to Saint Kitts, with twelve students.

Currently the Windsor campus contains six buildings on forty-two acres of land. The university enrollment was approximately 1,500 students as of October 2011. Windsor is accredited by the Board of St Kitts and Nevis, and listed in FAIMER International Medical Education Directory (IMED) and in the WHO's Avicenna Directory for medicine.

Xavier University College of Medicine (Aruba, www.xuson.com)

Xavier University School of Medicine (XUSOM) was founded in 2004 and is chartered by the government of Aruba. The campus itself is a renovated, modern facility with over 125,000 square feet of space. Xavier University School of Medicine is listed in the FAIMER International Medical Education Directory (IMED) and in the WHO's Avicenna Directory for medicine is also provisionally accredited by the CAAM-HP and ACCM. In 2015, Xavier University School of Medicine was approved by the Hashemite Kingdom of Jordan.

APPENDIX 4

Where Are These Caribbean Schools?

THE BUSINESS STRATEGY of the investors operating medical schools in the in the Caribbean was quite simple. Identify an island country and reach an agreement with the government that would allow the building of a private university. All these countries had weak economies highly dependent on agriculture and tourism, their industrial output minimal and exports limited. Several suffered with the collapse of the sugar and banana industry. These countries would benefit from investment that an educational enterprise that could create sorely needed jobs, mobilize the construction industry and allow for small business to open serving this new population of faculty and students. This in turn would increase internal consumption of services and products and bring new tax revenues. In return, the investors would negotiate substantial tax advantages.

They all followed the same strategy, negotiating with relatively new governments operating in a country with very limited diversification of their economy. A new school was beneficial to the island, and the result was a long-term agreement.

We will present a brief report on each of the countries so the reader gains an appreciation of where these schools are located.

Antigua and Barbuda

The population in 2015 is reported to be 92,436 (July 2015) and 32,000 people live in the capital city of Saint John's. During cruise season, major lines stop for a day and some originate from there.

Antigua's economy is reliant upon tourism, both European and American, Many hotels and resorts are located around the coastline and a number of charter sailing boats with very good quality marinas can be found. It offers excellent marinas with very good accommodations and marine services. Nelson Harbor is a great place for boat chartering.

The island's single airport is served by several major airlines that connect directly with several major cities in the United States and England.

American University of Antigua is a major medical school and is also a substantial contributors to the economy.

Aruba

Aruba is a Dutch Caribbean island off the coast of Venezuela. The capital is Oranjestad and the populations is 112,162. English, Dutch, and Spanish spoken alongside the local tongue, Papiamento. Discovered and claimed for Spain in 1499, Aruba was acquired by the Dutch in 1636. The last decade saw a boom in the tourism industry.

Aruba seceded from the Netherlands Antilles in 1986 and became a separate, autonomous member of the Kingdom of the Netherlands. Movement toward full independence was halted at Aruba's request in 1990.

Barbados

Barbados is the wealthiest and most developed country in the Eastern Caribbean and enjoys one of the highest per capita incomes in the region. Many embassies are situated there and serving all of the Eastern Caribbean. It has good educational facilities and its health care serves as a referral from other islands.

Banking and tourism are currently the pillars of the economy In the past, the economy was highly dependent on sugarcane. Offshore finance and information services are now important foreign exchange.

Resorts, beaches, outstanding golf courses, and excellent restaurants make it attractive to European tourism and, to a lesser extent, American tourism.

All major airlines connect Barbados with major cities, and the United States and two British airlines offer direct flights to London.

Dominica

Dominica was the last of the Caribbean islands to be colonized by Europeans, due chiefly to the fierce resistance of the native Caribs. France ceded possession to Great Britain in 1763, which colonized the island in 1805. Some three thousand Carib Indians still living on Dominica are the only pre-Columbian population remaining in the eastern Caribbean.

Dominica is a mountainous Caribbean island nation with 365 rivers and a thick rain forest. A volcanically heated, steam-covered Boiling Lake, which falls within Morne Trois Pitons National Park and is one of the hiking tourist attractions. The Boiling Lake is a major attraction and a very exciting hike The Trafalgar Falls represent another interesting and easy-to-reach tourist attraction.

The capital is Roseau, a city with an attractive waterfront. There are many villages along the Caribbean and Atlantic coast. The island population is 72,003 (2013) and has suffered significant emigration as a consequence of natural disasters and a fragile economy.

The Dominican economy has been dependent on agriculture—primarily bananas—in years past, but increasingly has been driven to tourism as the government seeks to promote Dominica as an ecotourism and an excellent diving destination. Hotels and restaurant industry need a lot of development. In 2009 and 2013, the economy contracted as a result of the global recession; growth remains anemic.

In 1978, in order to diversify the island's economy, the government opened its doors to offshore medical education that according to reports generates approximately one third of the country economy. It is also attempting to foster an offshore financial industry.

Ross University operates a medical school since 1978 and is one of the main pillars of the country's economy.

Transportation to Dominica is provided by air from San Juan Puerto Rico by Seaborne Airlines and by LIAT from Antigua and other Caribbean countries. Other minor airlines provide service to other islands. Dominica can also be reached by scheduled ferry services from Saint Lucia, Martinique, and Guadalupe. Air services from the United States have to be done through San Juan or Antigua, with limited number of flights a day.

Grenada

Carib Indians inhabited Grenada when Christopher Columbus discovered the island in 1498, but it remained uncolonized for more than a century. The French settled Grenada in the seventeenth century, established sugar estates, and imported large numbers of African slaves. Britain took the island in 1762 and vigorously expanded sugar production. In the nineteenth century, cacao eventually surpassed sugar as the main export crop. In the twentieth century, nutmeg became the leading export. In 1967, Britain gave Grenada autonomy over its internal affairs.

Full independence was attained in 1974, making Grenada one of the smallest independent countries in the Western Hemisphere. Grenada was seized by a Marxist military council on 19 October 1983. Six days later, the island was invaded by US forces and from six other Caribbean nations, They quickly captured the ringleaders and their hundreds of Cuban advisers. Newsworthy was the liberation of medical students at Saint George's University. Free elections were reinstituted the following year, and a democratic system has continued since then.

Grenada relies on tourism as its main source of foreign exchange especially since the construction of an international airport in 1985. Strong performances in construction and manufacturing, together with the development of tourism and higher education contributed to growth in national output; however, economic growth remained stagnant in 2010–14, after a sizable contraction in 2009, because of the global economic slowdown's effects on tourism and remittances.

The population is 110,000 living in the capital and other smaller villages.

Air transportation is through two major airports, and major US carriers reach Grenada nonstop from Miami, New York, and other major cities.

Saint George's University operates one of the best medical schools in the Caribbean and also has other degree-granting programs.

Saba

Saba, a Caribbean island in the Lesser Antilles chain, is a special municipality of the Netherlands. Measuring just thirteen square kilometers, it consists essentially of the top of the dormant Mount Scenery volcano. Its surrounding Saba Marine Park, a renowned dive site, is home to coral formations, dolphins, sharks, and turtles. There are also offshore seamounts, or underwater mountains created by volcanic activity.

The population is 1,824 (2010), and the island can be reached by air transportation via San Juan and is served by small Caribbean airline such as Air Antilles or Winair.

Sint Maarten

Sint Maarten, part of the Kingdom of the Netherlands, is a country on the southern part of a Caribbean island shared with Saint Martin, a French overseas collectivity. Natural landscapes span lagoons, beaches, and salt pans, while the capital, Philipsburg, has cobblestone streets and colorful, colonial-style buildings lining its Front Street shopping area. The port is a popular cruise-ship stop.

Saint Lucia

The island has its fine natural harbor at Castries. As several other Caribbean islands, Saint Lucia was disputed between England and France throughout the seventeenth and early eighteenth centuries (changing possession fourteen times); it was finally ceded to the UK in 1814.

Even after the abolition of slavery on its plantations in 1834, Saint Lucia remained an agricultural island, dedicated to producing tropical commodity crops. Self-government was granted in 1967 and independence in 1979, and it operates a progressive and efficient government working towards economic development. Its population is estimated at 182,000.

The island nation has been able to attract foreign business and investment, especially in its offshore banking and tourism industries. Tourism is Saint Lucia's main source of jobs and income—accounting for 65% of GDP—and the island's main source of foreign exchange earnings. The manufacturing sector is the most diverse in the eastern Caribbean area. Crops such as bananas, mangos, and avocados continue to be grown for export, but Saint Lucia's once-solid banana industry has been devastated by strong competition.

Its government policies has allowed for several medical schools to open including the following:

Spartan Health Sciences University
College of Medicine and Health Sciences
International American University (IAU)
American International Medical University (AIMU)
Caribbean Medical University (CMU)
Atlantic University School of Medicine (AUSOM)

Saint Vincent

Saint Vincent and the Grenadines is a southern Caribbean nation comprising a main island, Saint Vincent, and a chain of smaller ones. With yacht-filled harbors, chic private isles and volcanic landscapes, it's known for its major sailing destinations such as reef-lined Bequia Island. The main island is home to the capital, Kingstown.

Resistance by native Caribs prevented colonization on Saint Vincent until 1719. Disputed between France and the United Kingdom for most of the eighteenth century, the island was ceded to the latter in 1783. Between 1960 and 1962, Saint Vincent and the Grenadines was a separate administrative unit of the Federation of the West Indies. Autonomy was granted in 1969 and independence in 1979.

Success of the economy hinges upon seasonal variations in agriculture, tourism, and construction activity as well as remittance inflows. Much of the workforce is employed in banana production and tourism, but persistent high unemployment has prompted many to leave the islands. Saint Vincent is home to a small offshore banking sector and has moved to adopt international regulatory standards.

It is vulnerable to natural disasters. With estimated damage exceeding $110 million, tropical storms wiped out substantial portions of crops in 1994, 1995, and 2002. Heavy rainfall caused substantial damage to infrastructure, homes, and crops, which the World Bank estimated at US$112 million.

The government's ability to invest in social programs and respond to external shocks is constrained by its high public debt burden, which was 67% of GDP.

In 2013, the islands had more than 200,000 tourist arrivals, mostly to the Grenadines. The arrival numbers represented a marginal increase from 2012 but remain 26% below Saint Vincent's 2009 peak. Weak recovery in the tourism and construction sectors limited growth in 2015.

Air transportation to Saint Vincent and the Grenadines is through LIAT mainly from Antigua and Jet Blue from major US cities.

Saint Kitts

Saint Kitts and Nevis is a dual-island nation situated. It is known for cloud-shrouded mountains and beaches. Many of its former sugar plantations are now inns or atmospheric ruins. The larger of the two islands, Saint Kitts, is dominated by the dormant Mount Liamuiga volcano, home to a crater lake, green vervet monkeys, and rainforests crisscrossed with hiking trails.

Carib Indians occupied the islands of the West Indies for hundreds of years before the British began settlement in 1623. In 1967, the island territory of Saint Christopher-Nevis-Anguilla became an associated state of the UK with full internal autonomy. The island of Anguilla rebelled and was allowed to secede in 1971. The remaining islands achieved independence in 1983 as Saint Kitts and Nevis. In1998, a referendum on Nevis to separate from Saint Kitts fell short of the two-thirds majority vote needed. Nevis continues in its efforts to separate from Saint Kitts.

The economy of Saint Kitts and Nevis depends on tourism; since the 1970s, tourism has replaced sugar as the economy's traditional mainstay. Roughly 200,000 tourists visited the islands in 2009, but reduced tourism arrivals and foreign investment led to an economic contraction in 2009–2013, and the economy returned to growth only in 2014. Like other tourist destinations in the Caribbean, Saint Kitts and Nevis is vulnerable to damage from natural disasters and shifts in tourism demand.

Following the 2005 harvest, the government closed the sugar industry after several decades of losses. To compensate for lost jobs, the government has embarked on a program to diversify the agricultural sector and to stimulate other sectors of the economy, such as export-oriented manufacturing and offshore banking. The government has made notable progress on reducing its public debt, from 154% of GDP in 2011 to 83% in 2013, although it still faces one of the highest levels in the world, largely attributable to public enterprise losses.

As many other islands, Saint Kitts benefits of offshore education, and at the moment, the following institutions operate medical schools:

Medical University of the Americas
Windsor University School of Medicine
University of Medical Health Sciences (UMHS)

Air transportation to Saint Kitts is directly from major US Airlines from several major cities as well as direct flights to the UK.

BIBLIOGRAPHY

Federation of State Medical Boards. *2014 Physician Census.* https://www.fsmb.org/Media/Default/PDF/Census/2014census.pdf.

Accreditation Commission on Colleges of Medicine. www.accredmed.org.

Ahmadiyya Muslim Community USA. "The Ins & Outs of Caribbean Medical Education."

American Association of Medical Colleges. *2013 Physician Workforce Data Book.* American Association of Medical Colleges, 2013.

———. "Performance on Licensing Examinations." *2013 State Physician Workforce Data Book IV.*

———. *2015 State Physician Workforce Data Book.* Center for Workforce Studies.

———. *AAMC Data Book: Medical Schools and Teaching Hospitals by the Numbers (2016).*

———. Academic Medicine. US Medical School Matriculation by Gender. (Oct 2014) American Association of Medical Colleges. 2001–2014. Oct 2014.

———.*Graduation Rates and Attrition Factors for US Medical Students.* American Association of Medical Colleges, 2014.

———. *Applicants and Acceptees to US Medical Schools.* American Association of Medical Colleges, 2014.

———.aamc. Medical Students 1965–2013 American Association of Medical Colleges. 2001–2014. Oct 2014.

———. *Results of the 2014 Medical Education Enrollment Survey.* American Association of Medical Colleges, 2015.

aamc———. *Results of the 2014 Medical School Enrollment Survey. www.aamc.org*

m——. "Results of the 2015 Medical School Enrollment Survey." www.aamc.org.

———. *US Medical School Matriculation, 2001–2014.* American Association of Medical Colleges, 2014.

———. *US Medical Schools Matriculants, 2004–2014.*

American College of Physicians. *The Role of International Medical Graduates in the US Workforce: A Policy Monograph.* American College of Physicians, 2008.

American Medical Association. "IMGs in the United States." www.ama-assn.org.

———. *International Medical Graduates in the US Workforce Discussion.* American Medical Association, 2009.

Association of American Colleges. *US Medical School First Time Applicants.* Association of American Colleges, 2014.

BioMed Central. www.biomedcentral.com/1472-6920/10/5/prepub.

Caribbean Education Authority for Education in Medicine and Other Health Professions. www.caam-hp.org.

Caulfield, M., G. Redden, and H. Sondheimer. *Graduation Rates and Attrition Factors for US Medical Schools.* AAMC 13, no. 3 (May 2014).

Colby, S., and J. Ortman. *Projections of the Size and Composition of the US Population, 2014–2060.* US Census Bureau, US Department of Commerce.

Dahle, L. O., et al. "Pros and Cons of Vertical Integration between Clinical Medicine and Basic Science within a Problem-Based Undergraduate Medical Curriculum: Examples and Experiences from Linkoping, Sweden." *Med Teach* 24, no. 3 (2002): 280–285.

Davis, M. H., and R. M. Harden. "Planning and Implementing an Undergraduate Medical Education Curriculum: The Lessons Learned." *Medical Teacher* 25, no. 6 (2003): 596–608.

.www.caribbeanmedstudent.com.

Eckert, N. L., "Private Schools in the Caribbean: Outsourcing Medical Education." *Acad. Med.* 85 (2010): 622–30.

Eckert, N. L., and M. Van Zanten. *Overview of For-Profit Schools in the Caribbean.* FAIMER.

Farr, P. O. "The Impact of International Medical Graduates in US Health Care." *Mich. Med.* 105 (2006): 32.

Gastel, B. "Impact of International Medical Graduates on US and Global Health Care: Summary of the ECFMG 50th Anniversary Invitational Conference." *Acad. Med.* 81 (2006): S3–S6.

Glicksman, Eve. "Wanting It All: A New Generation of Doctors Places Higher Value on Work-Life Balance." *AAMC Reporter*, May 2013.

Government Accounting Office. Foreign Medical Schools: Educational Improve Monitoring of Schools that Participate in the Federal Student Loan Program 2010.

———. Foreign Medical Schools. Appendix IV. Performance on Licensing Examinations.

Hamilton, R., and E. Ramshaw. "State Can Permit Foreign Med Schools to Train in Texas." *The Texas Tribune*, Nov. 20, 2012.

"House, Senate Bills Address Foreign Medical School Access to Federal Student Loans." *Washington Highlights*, May 2015.

Institute of Medicine (US) Committee on the US Physician Supply. *The Nation's Physician Workforce: Options for Balancing Supply and Requirements.* Edited by Kathleen N. Lohr, Neal A. Vanselow, and Don E. Detmer. National Academies Press (US): 1996.

Johnson, D. G. "The AAMC Study of Medical Student Attrition: Overview and Major Findings." *J. Med. Education* 40, no. 10 (1965): 913–920.

Maher, B. M., H. Hynes, C. Sweeney, A. S. Kashan, M. O'Rourke. "Medical School Attrition—Beyond Statistics: A Ten-Year Retrospective Study." *BMC Med. Educ.* 13 (2013): 13.

Mc Nutt, D. "GMENAC: Its Manpower Forecasting Framework." *American Journal of Public Health* 71 (1981): 1116.

Moore, R.A., and E. J. Rhodenbaugh. "The Unkindest Cut of All: Are International Medical School Graduates Subjected to Discrimination by General Surgery Residency Programs?" *Curr. Surg.* 59 (2002): 228–236. doi: 10.1016/S0149-7944(01)00644-4.

Multpl.com. "US Population Growth Rate by Year." www.multpl.com/us population-growth-rate/table/by-year.

National Residency Matching Program. Charting Outcomes in the Match International Medical Graduates Characteristics of Applicants Who Matched to Their Preferred Specialty in the 2013

Main Residency Match. Jan 2014 NRMP. Advance data tables for 2016 Main Residency Match

Offshore Education in the OECS. Background paper prepared for the World Bank by Swedish Development Advisers. September 2004.

O'Neill, L., J. Hartvigsen, B. Wallstedt, L. Korsholm, and B. Eika. "Medical School Dropout—Testing at Admission versus Selection by Highest Grades as Predictors." Med. Educ. 45 (2011):1111–1120.

O'Riordan, Michael. "US Cardiologists in Short Supply, and the Problem Could Get Worse." *Medscape* 2009.

Pardes, H., and H. A. Pincus. "Report of the Graduate Medical Education National Advisory Committee and Health Manpower Development." *Arch. Gen. Psychiatry* 40, no. 1 (1983): 97–102.

Parsi, Kayhan. "International Medical Graduates and Global Migration of Physicians: Fairness, Equity, and Justice." *Medscape J Med.* 10, no. 12 (2008): 284.

Porter, Sheri. "Growing Shortage of Clinical Training Sites Challenges Medical Schools." *AAFP News,* July 6, 2014.

Riley, J. D, M. Hannis, and K. G. Rice. "Are International Medical Graduates a Factor in Residency Program Selection? A Survey of Fourth-Year Medical Students." *Acad. Med.* 71 (1996): 381–386. doi: 10.1097/00001888-199604000-00017.

Salsberg, Edward, and Atul Grover. "Physician Workforce Shortages: Implications and Issues for Academic Health Centers and Policymakers." *Academic Medicine* 81 (2006): 782–787.

Sandman, John. "This Is How Unqualified Doctor Wannabes Can Pay to Get Certified." *MainStreet,* December 19, 2013.

Schmidt, H. G. et al. "The Development of Diagnostic Competence: Comparison of a Problem-Based, an Integrated, and a Conventional Medical Curriculum." Acad. Med. 71 (1996): 658–64).

Smith, Mark. "Physician Supply: Surplus or Shortage?" *HealthLeaders Media,* January 17, 2008.

Staiger, D. O., D. I. Auerbach, and P. I. Buerhaus. "Trends in the Work Hours of Physicians in the United States." *JAMA* 303, no. 8 (2010): 747–53.

Staiger, D. O., and D. I. Auerbach. "Comparison of Physician Workforce Estimates and Supply." *JAMA* 30 (2009).

Start Medicine. www.startmedicine.com.

———. "Medical School Statistics." www.startmedicine.com/app/medstatistics.asp.

Stetto, J. E., G. D. Gacksetter, D. F. Cruess, and T. I. Hooper. "Variables Associated with Attrition from Uniformed Services University of the Health Sciences Medical School." *Mil. Med.* 169, no. 2 (2004): 1072–1075

Strayhorn, G. "Participation in a Premedical Summer Programme for Underrepresented Minorities as Predictor of Academic Performance in the First Three Years of Medical School: Two Studies." *Acad. Medicine* 74 (1999): 435–447.

Tinsely, J. A, and D. E. McAlpine. "Another Explanation for the Apparent Discrimination against International Medical Graduates by Residency Programs" (letter). *Am. J. Psych.* 156 (1999): 496–497.

"US Physician Supply and Requirements: Match or Mismatch?" *The Nation's Physician Workforce.* National Academic Press: 1996.

US Census Bureau. "US Population Growth by Year." US Census Bureau.

US Department of Health and Human Services–Health Resources and Services. *The Physician Workforce: Projections and Research into Current Issues Affecting Supply and Demand.* 2008.

Van Zanten, M., and J. R. Boulet. "Medical Education in the Caribbean: Quantifying the Contribution of Caribbean-Educated Physicians in the Primary Care Workforce." Acad. Med. 88 (2013) : 276–81.

———. "Medical Education in the Caribbean: Variability in Medical School Programs and Performance of Students." Academic Medicine 83 (2008): S33

"Where Do International Medical Graduates Fit in the US Healthcare Picture?" *Medscape Business of Medicine.* February 3, 2016.

Wikipedia.org. "List of Medical Schools in the Caribbean" https://en.wikipedia.org/wiki/List_of_medical_schools_in_the_Caribbean#Current_medical_schools_in_the_Caribbean.

Young, A., H. Chaudhry, J. Rhyne, and M. Dugan. "A Census of Actively Licensed Physicians in the United States, 2010." *Journal of Medical Education* 94 (2011): 50.

Zwyiak, W. *US Healthcare Workforce Shortages: Caregivers.*

www.ingramcontent.com/pod-product-compliance
Lightning Source LLC
Chambersburg PA
CBHW030932180526
45163CB00002B/543

* 9 7 8 1 5 2 4 5 3 3 6 2 5 *